Screening for Brain Impairment

A Manual for Mental Health Practice

Third Edition

Michael Franzen, PhD, was trained in clinical psychology at Southern Illinois University, and completed a clinical internship and a postdoctoral year of training in clinical neuropsychology at the University of Nebraska Medical Center. Dr. Franzen is currently Chief of Psychology/Neuropsychology and he serves as director of clinical internship training at Allegheny General Hospital in Pittsburgh, PA. He is an Associate Professor within the Department of Psychiatry and a faculty member of Drexel University College of Medicine. He has published widely in the field of clinical neuropsychology, and is actively involved in ongoing research. He is a Fellow of the American Psychological Association Division 40, the National Academy of Neuropsychology, and the Pennsylvania Psychological Association.

Glen Getz, PhD, received his doctorate in clinical psychology from the University of Cincinnati. Dr. Getz completed his internship and postdoctoral training in neuropsychology at Allegheny General Hospital, where he is currently a neuropsychologist conducting evaluations for both inpatients and outpatients. He is an Assistant Professor of Psychiatry at Drexel University College of Medicine. He has published in the field of clinical neuropsychology, and is actively involved in ongoing research. He is involved in training of undergraduate students, graduate students, clinical interns, psychiatry residents, child psychiatry fellows, and postdoctoral fellows in neuropsychology.

Screening for Brain Impairment

A Manual for Mental Health Practice

Third Edition

MICHAEL FRANZEN, PhD
GLEN GETZ, PhD

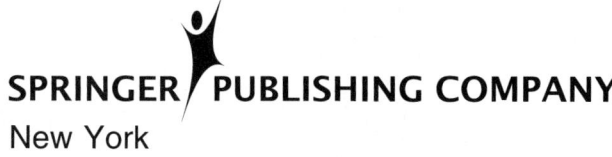

SPRINGER PUBLISHING COMPANY
New York

Copyright © 2010 Springer Publishing Company, LLC

All rights reserved.

No part of this publication may be reproduced, stored in a retrieval system, or transmitted in any form or by any means, electronic, mechanical, photocopying, recording, or otherwise, without the prior permission of Springer Publishing Company, LLC, or authorization through payment of the appropriate fees to the Copyright Clearance Center, Inc., 222 Rosewood Drive, Danvers, MA 01923, 978-750-8400, fax 978-646-8600, info@copyright.com or on the web at www.copyright.com.

Springer Publishing Company, LLC
11 West 42nd Street
New York, NY 10036
www.springerpub.com

Acquisitions Editor: Sheri W. Sussman
Senior Editor: Rose Mary Piscitelli
Cover design: David Levy
Composition: International Graphic Services

Ebook ISBN: 978-0-8261-1076-3

10 11 12 13/ 5 4 3 2 1

The author and the publisher of this Work have made every effort to use sources believed to be reliable to provide information that is accurate and compatible with the standards generally accepted at the time of publication. The author and publisher shall not be liable for any special, consequential, or exemplary damages resulting, in whole or in part, from the readers' use of, or reliance on, the information contained in this book. The publisher has no responsibility for the persistence or accuracy of URLs for external or third-party Internet Web sites referred to in this publication and does not guarantee that any content on such Web sites is, or will remain, accurate or appropriate.

Library of Congress Cataloging-in-Publication Data

Franzen, Michael D., 1954-
   Screening for brain impairment : a manual for mental health practice.—3rd ed / Michael Franzen, Glen Getz.
       p. ; cm.
   Rev. ed. of: Screening for brain impairment / Richard A. Berg, Michael Franzen, Danny Wedding. 2nd ed. c1994.
   Includes bibliographical references and index.
   ISBN 978-0-8261-1075-6 (alk. paper)
   1. Neuropsychological tests—Handbooks, manuals, etc. 2. Brain—Diseases—Diagnosis—Handbooks, manuals, etc. I. Getz, Glen. II. Berg, Richard (Richard A.). Screening for brain impairment. III. Title.
   [DNLM: 1. Neuropsychology—methods. 2. Cerebral Cortex—physiopathology. 3. Neuropsychological Tests. WL 103.5 F837s 2010]
   RC386.6.N48B47 2010
   616.8'0475—dc22
                                      2010008762

Printed in the United States of America by Hamilton Printing

This volume is dedicated to Debbie, Joe, Tim, and Rose, and to Dana, Maia, and Anna.

Contents

Preface		*ix*
Acknowledgments		*xiii*
1	Neurological Disorders	1
2	Psychiatric Disorders With Neurological Implications	31
3	Approaches to Neurological Assessment	41
4	The Neuropsychological History	55
5	The Mental Status Examination	75
6	Screening Tests of Perceptual and Motor Functions	103
7	Screening Tests for Verbal Functions	125
8	Screening Tests for Memory Functions	139
9	Screening Tests for Higher Cognitive Functions	153
10	Neuropsychological Screening	167
11	Effort and Motivation	185
12	Computerized Assessments	193
Glossary		199
References		213
Index		233

Preface

This book originally was, and this third edition still is, intended for the general clinician who is faced with the task of assessing clients who may or may not have organic impairment. It is not intended to provide the expertise needed to allow general clinicians to perform neurological or neuropsychological evaluations. Both of these evaluations require specialized didactic and experiential training that takes several years to acquire, and that cannot be replaced by reading this or any other book.

This book's current and previous authors are clinical psychologists with graduate training in behavioral medicine, neuropsychology, and additional specialized postdoctoral training in clinical neuropsychology. However, we are often called on to consult general clinicians who have to evaluate patients or clients whose problems may have questionable organic etiologies. It became apparent that there is a gap in the training of general clinicians, who are often not taught to recognize when referral to a specialist is appropriate.

Evaluation by a specialist, either a neurologist or a neuropsychologist, is an expensive endeavor, in terms of both money and time. Additionally, there are certain geographical areas where individuals may not have easy access to a specialist. There is, therefore, a particular need for a set of procedures that can be used by the general clinician, and that can focus the available information before a decision to refer is made.

Because this text was originally written several years ago, there has been a proliferation of new and updated assessment devices. We have made changes to reflect these new devices, as well as eliminate some of the older, less useful ones for which little new data have emerged. Sections on new issues, such as effort and motivation and use of computerized assessments, have been added, as well.

The primary goal of this book is to provide the clinician with procedures that can be used in the general outpatient clinical setting.

For the most part, the procedures described in this book can be used with a minimal investment in equipment.

A second goal of this book is to provide the general clinician with a translation of those terms and activities that are used by the specialist. The specialist has his own vocabulary, which can be useful when discussing conditions with other specialists, but which obfuscates the issues for the general clinician. Unfortunately, there is no certain method for ensuring that every specialist's report is written with plain diction, and in behavioral, rather than "foreign," terms. However, if the general clinician is armed with some knowledge of the language of specialists, she can derive more benefit from the referral report. The glossary that is provided at the end of this book should help the reader become more familiar with many of the technical terms and much of the jargon found in neurology and neuropsychology.

Not all of the procedures described in this book should be used with every patient. However, the procedures described here provide a useful outline for the evaluation of the patient with suspected central nervous system dysfunction. The first step is always to take a thorough history. The depth of history will vary from patient to patient. If information regarding the etiology of an organic problem surfaces during the history interview, that area should be followed up with a more intensive line of questioning. Of course, the direction pursued by the clinician taking the history will be determined, in part, by some understanding of the way in which various neurological disorders present clinically and across time. We will attempt to present this information succinctly in the first two chapters of this book.

If the history, clinical presentation, or referral of a patient suggests an organic etiology, then a mental status examination (MSE) should be conducted. The procedures in the chapter on the MSE can be used as a flexible guide to evaluation. The purpose of the MSE is to uncover additional information before a decision to refer is made. In no case should an MSE take the place of the complete neuropsychological and neurological evaluation.

There are three possible outcomes of the MSE. First, the MSE may not result in any indications of organic etiology, in which case, no referral is made. Second, the MSE may uncover some definite evidence of organic impairment, and the general clinician may decide to refer to a specialist. Third, the MSE may uncover only suggestions of impairment, in which case, the general clinician may want to investigate further the possibility of organic impairment before referring to a specialist. The chapters on screening instruments can be useful at this point. For example, if the history and MSE uncover suspected deficits in visual functioning, the general clinician can turn to the chapter on screening tests for perceptual and motor functions. On the basis of the patient's performance, a better decision to refer can be made.

There is yet another source of information that the clinician can use in deciding whether or not to refer, and that is the specialist herself. Often, the needed information is only a telephone call away. If the case does not involve an emergent condition, it would be better to send a copy of the MSE or screening results to the specialist. Naturally, these materials should not be sent without advance warning. The best situation would be one in which the general clinician has developed a working relationship with the specialist. We would also recommend that the general clinician be consumer-minded in the search for a specialist. Not all specialists are equal in skill or in the ability to provide useful information to the original referral source. The general clinician can give feedback to the specialist regarding the utility of the results and report, and can ask further questions that have not been addressed by the report. The specialist can be helped by being provided a complete history, along with a copy of the results of any evaluations conducted prior to referral. It also facilitates the process if the general clinician can provide a specific question in the referral request.

We hope this book will be useful to the general clinician. We believe it will prove helpful to both the practicing clinician and to graduate students, who can use it to learn more about cortical dysfunctions and to increase their personal repertoires of assessment techniques. Ultimately, we hope the book will lead to more accurate assessment and better treatment for the large number of patients who will be screened by clinicians who have read this book.

The feedback we have received on the book since the original publication has been gratifying, and indicates that our original goals of providing a useful resource for general clinicians and students have, in large measure, been met. We hope that this updated version will continue to prove to be a useful adjunct for clinicians.

Michael Franzen, PhD
Glen Getz, PhD

Acknowledgments

A number of people have helped us plan, develop, and communicate the ideas in this book. We are, of course, appreciative of Drs. Richard Berg and Danny Wedding, the coauthors of the previous editions. We are grateful to Sheri W. Sussman and Kerry Vegliando for their patience and editorial assistance. We thank our teachers, and we hope our own students learn as much from us. We thank Drs. P. V. Nickel and Anthony Mannarino for their support of our endeavors. We very much appreciate the creative efforts of Carol Stroud, who produced much of the original artwork without compensation and without complaining. Dr. Neha Thepa, Matthew Facciani, Jenna Dlugos, and Vanessa Vudy spent countless hours collecting research articles to update the book. Dana Getz and Debbie Franzen also helped us in numerous ways during the months devoted to researching and preparing this book. Finally, we wish to acknowledge the support and contribution of our families.

1 Neurological Disorders

Psychologists and other nonmedical mental health personnel routinely evaluate patients with psychiatric disorders. However, psychiatric disorders often coexist with neurological disorders; at other times, neurological disorders may present with classic psychiatric symptoms. Although neuropsychologists and psychiatrists are typically trained in differential diagnosis of these two classes of disorders, other mental health workers without special interest in brain functions often receive little or no training in how to assess the probability of brain disorders. They may be unaware of classic signs that signal cognitive impairment and indicate the need to refer to neurologists or other competent medical authorities.

In this chapter, we survey traditional neurodiagnostic categories, presenting what we believe to be the most essential facts that need to be remembered by all mental health personnel. We also review the types of neurodiagnostic data likely to be included in a patient's chart, so that the reader will be able to read and understand this sometimes cryptic information. We discuss the relevance of the mental status examination (MSE) and the patient's history, and, finally, we review the major screening techniques readily available to all psychologists to help identify those patients with likely brain disease.

BRAIN TUMORS

Patients with cerebral tumors are routinely seen in the neuropsychology laboratory, and they are not uncommon in general clinical practice. All psychologists should have a basic understanding of neoplastic disease, because the first signs of a brain tumor are often psychological, and tumor symptoms may mimic depression or anxiety. Depression and psychomotor slowing are commonly found to accompany cerebral impairment, and anxiety is a prominent feature of tumors in and around the third ventricle (Hall, 1980). Anxiety is said to increase as tumors progress. In addition, vague mental symptoms are often the only initial complaints of the patient with a cerebral lesion. Taylor (1982) states that some perceptible cognitive deficit occurs in 77% of brain tumor cases, confusion occurs in 59%, and disorientation occurs in approximately 40%.

Limbic system tumors mimic both schizophrenia and psychotic depression. They stand as an especially striking example of the importance of a thorough differential diagnosis and underscore the importance of at least a rudimentary understanding of brain disease for every psychologist. These links are briefly discussed in the next chapter as well.

Because psychologists are the point of entry into the health care system for many patients, it is critical that all psychologists be sensitive to the symptoms associated with intracranial tumors. Headaches are the most common single complaint of patients with brain tumors, and headaches will be present in about 60% of cases. Headaches will be the first sign of brain tumor in approximately 20% of cases (Reitan & Wolfson, 1985). The clinician's suspicion is raised when the patient reports that headaches are worse on arising in the morning, that they awaken him from sleep, or that they improve as the day progresses. Headaches associated with brain tumors tend to be exacerbated by coughing, sneezing, lifting, or straining to pass stools; they are often relieved when the patient lies down. The headaches are typically described as constant and nonpulsating, and dull and generalized.

Any history of projectile vomiting in adults increases the likelihood of organic disease, especially when the vomiting is not preceded by nausea and when the patient's headache improves after vomiting.

Seizures occur as a first symptom of tumors in approximately 15% of cases; they occur at some point in about 20–30% of all tumor cases (Strub & Black, 1988). The clinician should be especially suspicious when seizures develop in the adult in the absence of head trauma, alcoholism, or some obvious causal factor. Papilledema (swelling of the optic disc) is the result of increased intracranial pressure, and it can be readily observed with an ophthalmoscope. Papilledema can be an important sign of a brain tumor. Although psychologists typically lack the training and equipment necessary for a detailed ocular examination, it is good practice for psychologists to routinely examine the patient's eyes to check for ptosis, cranial nerve defects, and possible metabolic problems. In addition, it is important that all patients who present with any possibility of brain disease be asked about bowel and bladder function. Any report of increased sensitivity to the effects of drugs or alcohol should alert the clinician to the possibility of a brain tumor. The clinician should always seek medical evaluation for the patient who presents with signs of cognitive impairment in tandem with incontinence of recent onset. Further, consideration for referral to a neurologist or other specialist should also occur.

The clinical presentation of neoplastic disease can also include drowsiness, impaired judgment, memory loss, and altered mental functioning. Screening measures (discussed in chapters 6–12 of this book) can be especially helpful in providing data for decision making in these cases. Although symptoms will vary according to lesion type, location, and rate of growth, at least 50% of tumor cases will involve psychiatric symptoms. This is especially likely in the case of tumors involving the limbic system or the frontal or temporal lobes. Hallucinations may occur, along with other psychological symptoms such as depression, apathy, elation, loss of fundamental social skills, and subtle changes in personality. The general rule is that slow-growing tumors produce changes in personality and allow premorbid tendencies to manifest, more rapidly growing tumors lead to cognitive defects, the most rapidly growing lead to acute organic reactions with obvious impairment of consciousness (Lishman, 1978). The only early signs of a tumor may be the patient's torpid mental state, a mild slowing in behavioral response, a mild impairment on neuropsychological measures, and a characteristically long pause before answering questions. However, the brain is an astonishingly adaptable organ, and tumors that are sufficiently slow-growing may be totally asymptomatic or may produce such subtle signs that the change will be vaguely discerned by family members, but will be missed by all but the most perspicacious clinicians.

It is useful for the psychologist to be acquainted with the major methods of classifying tumors. First of all, tumors in the central nervous system (CNS) can be primary or secondary. Primary tumors are those that actually arise from cells within the CNS; secondary tumors arise in other areas of the body and spread or metastasize through the bloodstream to the brain and other organs. Approximately 15% of intracranial tumors are metastatic; usually, the original host site is the lung or the breast (Wiederholt, 1982). A total of 18% of patients who die from cancer will be shown at autopsy to have intracranial metastases (Adams & Victor, 1977). The prognosis for the patient with metastatic cancer is uniformly bleak, and patients who develop brain metastases typically live for only a few months. Neuropsychological evaluation of the patient with secondary brain metastatic lesions presents a spotty picture of weaknesses, with multiple pockets of dysfunction across the hemispheres.

Tumors are also sometimes classified as intrinsic or extrinsic. Intrinsic tumors develop from support cells within neural tissue; extrinsic tumors develop outside the brain, typically in the meninges. The most common example is the meningioma, a tumor that is usually slow-growing, developing between the skull and the brain. About 20% of intracranial tumors are meningiomas. They are easily identified with brain scans and they can usually be surgically resected. If the tumor is identified in time, the patient's prognosis is good. Mental functions are affected by the pressure exerted by the space-occupying properties of the meningioma, and sometimes by erosion of the surrounding neural tissue. Neuropsychologically, the meningioma presents a less lateralized picture, and it rarely produces suppressions. (Suppressions refer to the failure to perceive a stimulus on one side with bilateral simultaneous stimulation. Suppressions can be auditory, visual, or tactile, and are commonly seen with intrinsic tumors.) In addition, in the case of meningiomas, the psychologist is less likely to observe the striking differences between verbal and performance IQ values that are common with intrinsic tumors. Middle-aged women appear to be at especially high risk for developing meningiomas (Bubb, 1984).

Brain tumors can be classified as *benign* or *malignant*, depending on the rapidity of growth of the tumor and the likelihood of spread to surrounding tissue. About 40% of brain tumors are benign; however, this distinction is of less value in the case of neural neoplasms, insofar as any tumor that invades the cranial vault is dangerous and potentially lethal. Lethality is rated on a graduated scale, with Grade I neoplasms the least dangerous, and Grade IV neoplasms the most dangerous.

Finally, tumors can be meaningfully classified by type, according to the nature of the original cell from which they derive. Gliomas, for example, arise from glial cells, the connective tissue of the brain. Gliomas are the most common form of brain tumor and comprise approximately 50% of intracranial tumors, often lethal. Subtypes of gliomas include the highly lethal glioblastoma multiforme, astrocytomas, ependymomas, oligodendrogliomas, and medulloblastomas. The glioblastoma multiforme is the most common form, comprising about 50% of gliomas. These lesions occur most frequently in men between the ages of 40 and 60. Because most cases of glioblastoma develop from astrocytes, some writers refer to glioblastomas as astrocytomas, Grade III or IV.

In general, children are more likely to develop tumors arising in the *brainstem* and *cerebellum*, whereas primary tumors in the cerebral cortex are more common in adults. The clinical presentation of tumors is more variable in children, and it is more difficult to predict how a neoplasm will affect function in the developing brain. Even in the adult, because localization of some lesions may be difficult, bilateral or diffuse dysfunction can result from pressure effects and edema.

VASCULAR DISORDERS

Blood supplies the brain with oxygen and glucose and disposes of heat and metabolic wastes; disruption of regular blood flow to specific brain areas for more than a few minutes will almost always result in damage to the neural tissue surrounding the damaged vessel. Fortunately, there is redundancy in the complexity of cerebral vascularity, and collateral circulation can often provide blood to a region of the brain when it is cut off from its normal supply.

Cerebrovascular accidents (CVAs) are also referred to as apoplexy or strokes. CVAs represent a public health problem of enormous proportions. CVAs are the third leading cause of death in the United States, and costs related to stroke reached up to $62.7 billion in 2007 (American Heart Association Statistics Committee, 2007). Approximately 795,000 people suffer strokes each year in the United States (American Stroke Association, 2009). Of these, 10% will die immediately, and 20–40%

will die in the months following a stroke. Of the survivors, 10% will be totally disabled and will have to be institutionalized; 40% will require nursing care; 40% will have a persistent, mild neurological defect; and only 10% will totally recover. Nearly 1/4 of the people who suffer stroke are under the age of 65. It is the rare individual whose life or family has not been affected in some way by vascular disease. For those who do recover, improvement will typically follow a decelerating learning curve, with the most improvement noted in the first 6 months, and with physical disabilities typically resolving more quickly than cognitive defects.

The occurrence of a CVA is almost always preceded by the process of atherosclerosis, in which arteries become hardened and clogged with yellowish-white layers of cholesterol. This gradual stenosis (progressive narrowing of the cerebral vessels) at some point may totally occlude blood flow. Carotid endarterectomy, a surgical technique for cleaning the vessels carrying blood to the brain, is sometimes helpful in reestablishing blood supply.

Epidemiological research has isolated the major risk factors for stroke. Increasing age and hypertension stand alone as the two best individual predictors of cerebrovascular disease. Systolic pressure is a slightly better predictor than diastolic. However, atherosclerosis, diabetes, rheumatic heart disease, smoking, hypercholesterolemia, and use of birth control pills are also major predictors, as are race and sex (African Americans have more strokes than Whites, and men have more strokes than women). In addition, a person with a history of a CVA is at least 10 times as likely (as the average person of his age and sex) to have another stroke. The process of atherosclerosis is intimately linked to behavior, habit, and lifestyle, and it becomes increasingly clear that there is nothing "accidental" about CVAs.

A basic understanding of vascular anatomy is essential for understanding cerebrovascular disease. The brain is supplied bilaterally by the internal carotid arteries and the vertebral arteries. The internal carotid divides on each side to form the anterior and middle cerebral arteries. The vertebral arteries form a single basilar artery, which divides at the top of the midbrain to form paired posterior cerebral arteries. The posterior cerebral arteries supply blood to the thalamus, the occipital lobes, and the medial temporal lobes. The entire system is linked by the Circle of Willis and by the anterior and posterior communicating arteries, providing for collateral circulation.

Most strokes occur in the region of the middle cerebral artery. This region serves major motor and sensory areas around the Rolandic fissure, accounting for the paralysis and sensory deficits that often accompany a stroke. A stroke in the middle cerebral artery is likely to produce contralateral weakness (with the arms and face weaker than the leg), contralateral sensory loss, homonymous hemianopsia, and dementia. If the dominant hemisphere is involved, an expressive aphasia is likely to result. Middle cerebral artery strokes on the right side will frequently produce denial of defects (anosognosia). Left-sided neglect is also common in these cases. If the stroke affects gaze on either side, the eyes will tend to "look" toward the side of the lesion.

Wolf (1980) has observed that total occlusion of the middle cerebral artery is more lethal in younger patients than in the elderly, because in old age, there has been sufficient cerebral atrophy to ensure that the cerebral edema that accompanies a middle cerebral artery stroke does not cause an abrupt rise in intracranial pressure or herniation and brainstem compression.

Anterior cerebral artery infarcts are less likely to occur than middle cerebral artery strokes, and may produce contralateral weakness in the leg (although sparing the arm), contralateral sensory loss, dementia, urinary incontinence, and an affective disturbance. In addition, primitive grasp and sucking reflexes may be produced on the contralateral side.

Posterior cerebral artery infarcts are also relatively rare, but they produce fascinating clinical phenomena. Memory impairment is often present, especially when there is temporal lobe involvement. Contralateral visual field cuts will occur with damage to the calcarine cortex. Alexia without agraphia is common when the damage is to the dominant occipital lobe along the posterior corpus callosum. Bilateral posterior cerebral infarcts will often lead to cortical blindness with personal denial of disability. This form of anosognosia is called *Anton's syndrome*. In general, posterior strokes are far more likely to produce bilateral signs of damage. If the stroke is low enough to affect the reticular formation, loss of consciousness and eventual death will result.

CVAs can be conveniently (if not precisely) categorized as either infarcts (occlusions) or hemorrhages. The former is more common by a ratio of about 3 to 1; however, the hemorrhage is a far more serious neurological event and is lethal about four times as often as the infarct (Lishman, 1978).

Infarcts or obstructive strokes can be further subdivided into thrombotic or embolic subtypes. A *thrombus* occurs as the result of the accumulation of arteriosclerotic plaques, usually at the bifurcation of a vessel. The thrombus typically develops slowly and may be preceded by transient ischemic attacks (TIAs). Hypertension, diabetes, and smoking are all important risk factors for the development of thrombotic infarcts, which typically occur during sleep, probably because of the mild state of hypotension present when the patient is supine and sleeping. Thrombotic occlusions are more common than embolic ones.

The embolus is a fatty deposit that has broken away from a blood vessel wall, or, less commonly, a fragment of a thrombotic lesion that floats through the bloodstream until it becomes lodged in a vessel, blocking the passage of blood and producing *ischemia*. The onset of the embolic stroke is sudden; there are no warning signs. Headache is usually absent immediately after the stroke, and resolution, if it occurs, is rapid.

Hemorrhages are extremely serious neurological emergencies that result from blood spilling from a vessel and destroying surrounding brain tissue. Blood is often released under considerable pressure, and the eventual outcome of a particular stroke may be a function of whether or not blood is released away from or toward the brain itself. The onset of the hemorrhage is typically sudden and may be induced by physical exertion. Unlike thrombotic strokes, hemorrhages rarely occur during sleep. Severe headaches and loss of consciousness are the most common initial symptoms. Neuropsychological assessment of the patient who has had a cerebral hemorrhage almost always reveals suppressions and a strongly lateralized pattern of deficits.

Parsons (1983) has provided an analogy that can be used for appreciating the different varieties of traumatic hemorrhages—extradural, subdural, subarachnoid, and intracerebral. One needs first to remember that the brain is surrounded by a series of protective coverings—the meninges. At birth, there are only two membranes: the pia arachnoid, which adheres closely to the brain, and the dura, which is attached to the skull. The arachnoid eventually separates from the pia, but remains connected to it by a weblike process that forms the subarachnoid space. Parsons suggests that the student imagine that the brain was sprayed with a protective coat (the pia), wrapped in a sheet of foam rubber to prevent jolting (the arachnoid), sealed in a polyethylene bag (the dura), and then suspended from the roof of a very sturdy container (the skull) by a series of threads (the veins running to the sagittal sinus). An extradural hemorrhage occurs when the outer container fractures and a skull shard ruptures a meningeal artery. Blood promptly flows into the epidural space. Patients may recover briefly following an injury of this sort, but they relapse quickly as intracranial pressure rises. The pupil on the affected side becomes dilated and fixed, and there is a contralateral hemiparesis. Immediate neurosurgical intervention is required.

The subdural hematoma is an equally serious hemorrhage that occurs following relatively minor injuries (that may be so trivial as to go either unreported or unremembered). Following the Parsons analogy, the subdural hematoma occurs when one of the veins that suspend the brain from the sagittal sinus is ruptured. Blood gradually accumulates between the dura and the arachnoid layer, and symptoms may not develop until hours or days after the traumatic event. The clinician who works with the elderly and with alcoholics should be sensitive to the fact that subdural hematomas are especially frequent in both of these groups, and that computed tomography (CT) scans can be normal in as many as 10% of cases of subdural hematoma (Parsons, 1983). It is also important to remember that chronic subdural hematomas are more likely to impair consciousness and are less likely to affect movement, sensation, or vision, because most of their effect results from pressure rather than from specific neural destruction. In the patient who presents with marked clouding of consciousness or who is in a coma without severe hemiparesis, a subdural hematoma is a far more likely possibility than an ischemic stroke (Wolf, 1980). The subarachnoid hemorrhage accounts for 5–10% of strokes, and happens when bleeding occurs beneath the arachnoid layer. It is characterized by intense headaches and neck stiffness, and by the presence of blood in the cerebrospinal fluid (CSF). The hemorrhage can result from trauma; more often, it results from the bursting of an aneurysm (a congenital weakness in a vessel wall) or from an arteriovenous malformation (a congenital deformity in a vessel). The aneurysm could "balloon" and produce pressure effects. This results in an increased risk of rupturing because of the increased fragility of the vessel wall. An aneurysm that has not ruptured may be asymptomatic, but will typically produce localized neuropsychological deficits, with a low Impairment Index on the Halstead-Reitan Battery (Golden, 1981). Signs of a ruptured aneurysm include nausea, vomiting, and headaches. Berry aneurysms, so named because of their berrylike shape, are small, thin-walled aneurysms typically found at the bifurcation of vessels.

The psychologist will typically not see patients who have hemorrhaged, at least not in the acute state, but he or she will encounter patients who are having TIAs. TIAs are temporary reductions in blood supply to the brain, which, by definition, cannot last for more than 24 hours. They do not result in the death of neural tissue, but they do produce clinical signs, and they increase the likelihood that the patient will develop more serious cerebrovascular disorders. Twenty-five to 40% of patients with TIAs will have cerebral infarcts within 5 years; this incidence is 10 times that of people of the same age and sex in the general population (Olsen, Brumback, Gascon, & Christoferson, 1981).

The symptoms of a TIA will vary, depending on whether the carotid artery or the vertebrobasilar system is involved. In general, the symptoms of a TIA include vertigo, dysarthria, ataxia, vomiting, headaches, visual disturbances, motor or sensory loss, agraphia, and confusion. Although, historically, TIAs have been thought to produce little cognitive damage, closer analysis with neuropsychological testing reveals that mild cognitive impairment is found in these patients prior to the development of actual infarcts (Lezak, Howieson, & Loring, 2004).

When a vascular disorder is suspected, the clinician should always expand the history and inquire about visual disturbances and the presence of relevant risk factors, such as hypertension and oral contraceptives. In addition, the presence of crossed neurological signs (e.g., monocular blindness and contralateral hemiparesis or right-sided facial weakness with left hemiparesis) is strongly suggestive of vascular disease. It is important to appreciate that vascular disease can mimic endogenous depression; this is especially common in collagen vascular disease, such as systemic lupus erythematosus (Lechtenberg, 1982). These patients will often respond to treatment with antidepressant medication.

One frequent consequence of stroke is impaired circulation of the CSF. This can produce normal pressure hydrocephalus, characterized by a classic triad of clinical signs: dementia, gait disturbance, and urinary incontinence. Any patient presenting this constellation of symptoms should be referred at once for medical, and preferably neurological, evaluation. Treatment usually involves shunting CSF fluid from the lateral ventricles into the general circulation. Because the cause of the disorder is unknown, it is sometimes referred to as *occult hydrocephalus*. The peak age of onset is in the late fifties.

THE DEMENTIAS

The patient with a dementing illness is, in the most real and terrifying sense of the phrase, losing his mind. The term "dementia" refers to a clinical syndrome in which there is loss of brain function because of diffuse organic brain disease. It is a general term, but still somewhat more precise than the vague phrase "organic brain syndrome."

The dementias are characterized by insidious onset, dysfunction that is localized primarily in the cerebral hemispheres, demonstrable pathological changes in cerebral tissue, and the presence of memory loss as a common primary initial concern. Some writers define dementias as disorders that are irreversible; however, the more general current practice is to include a variety of conditions (e.g., Cushing's syndrome, nutritional deficiencies, Wilson's disease, etc.) that can be treated, with a potential reversal of the clinical signs of dementia. Table 1.1 lists the major causes of dementia. Schamhorst (1992) has proposed a useful mnemonic for remembering the most common reversible causes of dementia. This mnemonic is listed in Table 1.2.

The problem of dementia is becoming a public health concern of unparalleled dimension as the lifespan of the typical American continues to expand. Half of the U.S. population currently lives to at least the age of 75, and one fourth live to the age of 85. However, with increasing age, each of us is at increasing risk for developing a dementing illness, because 4–5% of people over the age of 65 have a moderate to severe dementia. The average lifespan from the time of diagnosis to death is slightly more than 7 years, with considerable variation across patients (Strub & Black, 1988). Although healthy lifestyle decisions have been suggested to prevent or slow the progression, there is no compelling evidence that dementia can be prevented through vascular manipulation or any behavioral means (Stephan & Brayne, 2008).

Alzheimer's disease is the single most common cause of dementia, accounting for approximately 50% of cases. There were fewer than 5.3 million cases of probable Alzheimer's disease in 2009, with about 5.1 million cases in those 65 years or older (Alzheimer's Association, 2009). Caring for these patients will require prodigious resources. The *current*

Table 1.1

MAJOR CAUSES OF DEMENTIA

Degenerative diseases of the CNS

    Alzheimer's disease

    Pick's disease

    Huntington's chorea

    Parkinson's disease

    Progressive supranuclear palsy

Vascular disorders

    Multi-infarct dementia

    Arteriovenous malformation

    Carotid artery occlusive disease

    Subarachnoid hemorrhage

    Cerebral embolism

    Binswanger's disease

Metabolic, endocrine, and nutritional disease

    Hypothyroidism and hyperthyroidism

    Hypocalcemia and hypercalcemia

    Hepatic failure

    Wilson's disease

    Renal failure

    Dialysis encephalopathy

    Cushing's syndrome

    Hypopituitarism

    Electrolyte disturbances

    Wernicke-Korsakoff syndrome

    Vitamin deficiency (especially B_1, B_6, B_{12}, niacin, folate)

Table 1.1 *(continued)*

Intracranial space-occupying lesions
Head trauma
Epilepsy
Infections
    Meningitis
    Encephalitis
    Syphilis
    Creutzfeldt-Jacob disease
    Kuru
    Multifocal leukoencephalopathy
Toxins and drugs
    Alcohol
    Drugs (prescription and nonprescription)
    Heavy metals (arsenic, lead, mercury, thallium)
    Carbon monoxide
    Organic solvents
Miscellaneous
    Multiple sclerosis
    Muscular dystrophy
    Normal pressure hydrocephalus

cost of Alzheimer's to the U.S. economy is $148 billion, with 9.9 million unpaid caregivers. These costs are bound to increase in the future.

Alzheimer's disease is a disorder that strikes females almost three times as often as males, likely associated with increased life expectancy in females. It has been associated historically with cognitive changes secondary to atherosclerosis. However, it appears that the cerebral vasculature plays a relatively minor role in the changes typically observed in these patients. Although pathophysiology of the disorder is not clearly understood, the brains of patients at autopsy have been shown to contain numerous senile plaques, neurofibrillary tangles, and Hirano bodies.

Table 1.2

MNEMONIC FOR COMMON REVERSIBLE CAUSES OF DEMENTIA

Drugs or alcohol use

Emotional disorders

Metabolic or endocrine disorders

Eye and ear dysfunctions

Nutritional deficiencies

Trauma, tumors, or toxins (e.g., lead poisoning)

Infections

Arteriosclerotic complications of the heart and brain

Genetic studies have linked apolipoprotein E, complement receptor 1 (CR1), and PICALM. There is also marked degeneration of nerve cells. Although there is a slight increase in neuronal loss (about 5% per year greater than would be expected from aging effects alone), the dramatic atrophy sometimes observed on brain scans appears to be secondary to the shrinkage of neurons and loss of dendritic spines, rather than to simple loss of neurons (Wolf, 1980). Neuronal shrinkage is most prominent in the association areas of the cortex, and there is relative sparing of the sensory and motor cortex in the early stages of the illness. The severity of symptoms will correlate directly with the mass of tissue lost, the density of senile plaques and neurofibrillary tangles, and the degree of ischemic softening present. Although this process is pathological in the case of Alzheimer's disease, by the tenth decade of life, virtually every human brain is found to contain senile plaques and tangles.

Wells and Duncan (1980) have delineated three characteristic stages in the progression of dementia. In the early stage, there are multiple vague symptoms that are often diagnosed as functional. There are multiple somatic complaints that do not fit easily identifiable patterns. Complaints of weakness, insomnia, constipation, and dizziness are common, as are depression and irritability. There is apt to be confusion in response to very slight provocation (e.g., a change in appointment times), and this behavior is usually inconsistent with premorbid personality. The patient will frequently make excuses for poor performance ("I've never been very good at math"). *Memory deficits are especially common and will frequently be the chief complaint.* Patients find that they have to struggle to complete what used to be easy tasks, and they may make excessive use of notes, lists, and schedules. *It is rare for the medical/ neurological evaluation of the patient to be positive in the early phase of the illness; however, cognitive deficits will typically be apparent on neuropsychological screening.* Neuropsychological findings will prove most valuable when they are inconsistent with educational or vocational history.

It is important to appreciate that many patients become quite good at rationalizing their failures. Friends and coworkers may deliberately conspire to cover up the mistakes and mishaps of the patient. One of the authors once saw a patient who was clearly demented but who continued to go to work each day; on questioning, the patient acknowledged that he was "pretty much carried by my union brothers." Patients may also cope with their loss of cognitive skills by deferring to other family members during questioning, and by claiming that the questions or the testing procedures being employed are foolish and a waste of time. When neuropsychological screening does occur, motor skills and attention are apt to be found to be intact, and intellectual skills as measured by the *Wechsler Adult Intelligence Scale–Revised* (WAIS-R; Wechsler, 1987) are likely to be relatively well preserved in contrast to performance on more sensitive screening tests, such as Trails B and the Category Test.

In the middle phase of the dementia process, the patient's difficulties with orientation, memory, judgment, and problem solving become apparent, even with a rudimentary MSE. Mood is apt to be flat or labile, and there is typically diminished concern for appearance and personal hygiene. There are clear changes in personality and behavior. Primitive reflexes may emerge, and the psychologist may find it valuable to systematically test for abnormal reflexes. In the patient with primitive reflexes, a grasp reflex can be elicited simply by lightly stroking the patient's hand. A rooting reflex may be elicited by stroking the corners of the patient's mouth to see whether he turns his lips toward the stimulus. This response is normal in infants. A snout reflex will be demonstrated by the puckering of the patient's lips in response to gentle tapping on the lower lip with a pencil. Finally, a palmomental reflex will be observed in some demented patients. This occurs when the patient retracts one side of his mouth and chin in response to gentle stroking of his palm.

The psychologist will have little to contribute to assessment of the patient in the late phase of dementia. This phase is characterized by profound apathy and personality disturbance, with impairment of all mental, motor, and sensory abilities. By this stage, the patient is frequently bedfast, and will typically be incontinent for both urine and feces. Brain mass and weight are reduced, and there is often a global aphasia.

In the early stages of Alzheimer's disease, it is common for both the electroencephalogram (EEG) and the magnetic resonance imaging (MRI) scan to remain normal. With progression of the disease, the EEG will typically display mild diffuse slowing, whereas in many cases, the MRI scan will come to show ventricular enlargement and widening of the cortical sulci. There are decreases in both cerebral oxygen uptake and cerebral blood flow.

The *WAIS-IV* is not especially sensitive to early dementias. If it is given, the psychologist will typically find that performance scores are lower than verbal scores. The *Wechsler Memory Scale–IV* (Wechsler, 1987) is apt to be more sensitive to the cognitive changes seen in dementia than is the *WAIS-IV*, and one would expect to find memory quotients lower than full-scale IQ scores. There is frequently considerable subtest scatter across the *WAIS* scales. Screening measures such as Halstead's Category Test and Part B of the Trail Making Test are likely to indicate clear cognitive impairment (Strub & Black, 1988). Mild dysnomia is frequently evident in patients with an early dementia, and tests of verbal fluency (such as the Controlled Word Association Test) may prove to be especially sensitive (Cummings, 1985).

Table 1.1 lists many disorders that can potentially be treated if identified. It is especially tragic when a patient with a reversible illness (normal pressure hydrocephalus, for example) is misdiagnosed as having Alzheimer's disease and is sent to a nursing home, when a correct diagnosis and appropriate treatment could have alleviated the symptoms that were present.

Pick's disease is a currently untreatable degenerative dementia that must ultimately be differentiated from Alzheimer's disease on the basis of histological findings. It is one fifth as common as Alzheimer's, and tends to affect the cerebral hemispheres differentially, producing more damage in the frontal and anterior temporal lobes (unlike Alzheimer's, which is characterized by more parietofrontal and hippocampal involvement). Because of the strong frontal involvement, patients with Pick's disease lose social graces early in the progression of the disease, and disinhibition is common. Many of these patients will develop echolalia. The Pick's patient is somewhat less likely to develop a seizure disorder, but is more likely than the Alzheimer's patient to develop signs of the Kluver-Bucy syndrome (orality, hyperphagia, hypersexuality, placidity, and sensory agnosia).

Repeated vascular occlusions or small hemorrhages can produce a multi-infarct dementia that is almost always accompanied by a history of hypertension. The neuropsychological picture is characterized by rapid onset with a more stepwise pattern of deterioration. The neurological and behavioral signs associated with multi-infarct dementias are more dramatic than those found with an Alzheimer's patient, but memory is likely to be better preserved in the multi-infarct patient. In addition, the patient with vascular disease is more likely to develop a pseudobulbar state (e.g., prolonged and exaggerated laughing or crying). In contrast to Alzheimer's, the patient with a multi-infarct dementia is slightly more likely to be male.

A number of other degenerative diseases can produce the syndrome of dementia. We can only mention a few of the more important ones here; however, more detailed descriptions are available in any standard neurology textbook.

Although James Parkinson believed there was no cognitive decline with the disease that today bears his name, evidence suggests he was wrong; although it is mild, there is an unquestionable dementia present in at least half of patients with Parkinson's disease (Lechtenberg, 1982). Specific neuropsychological deficits can be demonstrated in over 90% of patients with Parkinson's disease when appropriate tests are used (Cummings, 1985). Deficits tend to be in the areas of orientation, constructional abilities, and memory, with social behavior and language relatively spared. Executive functioning impairment in these patients may increase the likelihood for future dementia (Dujardin, Defebvre, Grunberg, Becquet, & Destée, 2004).

The most salient symptoms of Parkinson's disease are bradykinesia (slowness of movement), rigidity, and a resting tremor. In addition, the clinician should look for a masklike and expressionless face, diminished blinking, poor posture and balance, a shuffling gait, and the presence of involuntary "pill-rolling" movements. Micrographia is also frequently present. These patients are often clinically depressed, and may be taking antidepressant medication along with L-dopa. Psychiatric symptoms commonly develop in response to the necessary medication regimen.

Parkinson's disease results from loss of the capacity to produce dopamine in the basal ganglia. Parkinson's disease can be idiopathic, postencephalitic, or drug induced. It typically affects people over the age of 50. Men develop Parkinson's disease slightly more often than women.

Dementia is also a characteristic feature of Huntington's chorea, another basal ganglia disorder, which causes selective destruction in the caudate and putamen. The disease is an autosomal-dominant disorder, with onset of symptoms typically in the age range of 35–50 years. There is no difference between the rate of men and women who have Huntington's chorea.

Unfortunately, many victims of Huntington's disease have already had children by the time their disease is diagnosed. Fifty percent of these children will also develop the disorder. A positive family history is the single best predictor of Huntington's chorea. Genetic testing can determine whether chromosome 4 is mutated, consisting of expanded and unstable CAG trinucleotide repeat.

The movement disorder that accompanies Huntington's disease involves both chorea (brief, nonrepetitive jerks of the fingers, extremities, face, and trunk) and athetosis. Athetosis refers to the inability to sustain a particular group of muscles in one position because of interruption by slow, purposeless movements. In Huntington's disease, flexion of the wrist with extended fingers is especially common. The combination of athetosis and chorea of all four limbs is a cardinal feature of Huntington's chorea. However, in the early stages of the disorder, the clinician may miss subtle signs, which the patient frequently disguises by making the movement appear voluntary (e.g., brushing his hair back). We recommend asking the patient simply to sit still with his arms outstretched and his eyes shut; if it is present, the movement disorder should be apparent in this condition. Other motor problems can include facial grimacing, swaying, and lurching of gait. The movement disturbances frequently are exacerbated by stress and disappear with sleep.

Cognitive and personality changes frequently precede the development of movement disorders. Unlike many other dementias, the patient with Huntington's disease is acutely aware of his failing mental powers. This may contribute to the very high suicide rate that is present in these patients. In rare cases, onset of symptoms may begin in childhood or adolescence; early onset generally predicts a more rapid and severe deterioration. Death usually occurs within 15 years after the onset of the disease.

Multiple sclerosis (MS) should be mentioned along with the other dementias we have discussed, because it is important in the differential diagnosis of a variety of neurological disorders, and because in rare cases, dementia may be the initial presenting symptom. MS is a chronic degenerative disease, which typically destroys myelin in the white matter of the brain and spinal cord. The disorder strikes women more often than men, and it usually first presents between the ages of 20 and 40 (Kurtzke & Wallin, 2000). The disorder is quite rare before age 10 or after age 50. It occurs with greater frequency in individuals who reside in colder climates, and several studies suggest that people who migrate in childhood from colder climates carry an increased risk, even though the disease may not become apparent until 20 years or more after their migration.

MS is characterized by an unpredictable course with irregular exacerbations and remissions. Exacerbations may be triggered by stress, fatigue, temperature change, poor health, or menstruation. Primary presenting symptoms include weakness or numbness in one of the legs; a variety of visual disturbances, including diplopia; loss of visual acuity and visual field defects; brainstem defects such as vertigo and vomiting; gait disturbance; and disorders of micturition. Patients also sometimes display inappropriate affect, including euphoria and eutonia (a general feeling of pervasive physical well-being). Scanning speech (slowed speech with pauses between each syllable), along with tremor and nystagmus, are sometimes found (these three signs are referred to as Charcot's triad); however, it is critical for the clinician to appreciate that there are no truly typical presenting signs and symptoms in MS; it must be considered as part of the differential diagnosis with every patient who presents with a confusing clinical picture. Ultimately, the diagnosis has to be made on the basis of history, although some patients may have CSF abnormalities, pale optic discs, and clear abnormalities on visual, auditory, or somatosensory evoked potentials. Although not foolproof, MRI can aid in diagnosing MS, as it can detect central nervous system demyelination, MS plaques, and hyperintensities (Miller, 2003).

Wilson's disease, also known as hepatolenticular degeneration, is an autosomal recessive genetic disorder of copper metabolism. Genetic testing has implicated chromosome 13. It appears primarily in childhood and early adulthood. Although it can occur at any age, its first appearance is rare after age 35. There is no difference between men and women in frequency. It presents in many ways like Huntington's disease. However, Wilson's disease is a classic masquerader: at least 20% of cases will initially present solely with psychiatric symptoms such as anxiety, depression, mania, or paranoid thinking. These patients are often treated initially by a psychiatrist or psychologist.

The suicide rate for patients with Wilson's disease is quite high. It is critical that all psychologists be alert to the possibility of the disorder, because early treatment can reverse much of the damage that may have occurred. Treatment involves use of a chelating agent, such as penicillamine, to lower serum copper levels and increase urinary copper excretion. Prognosis is good with early identification. Without treatment, there is continuing loss of neurons in both the cortex and basal ganglia and increasing dystonia and dysarthria. Additional clinical signs of the disorder include the presence of a Kayser-Fleischer ring (a brown-green ring around the cornea that is pathognomonic for the disease), increased pigmentation of the anterior aspects of the lower legs, and blue-green lines running transversely across the fingernails.

Human Immunodeficiency Virus Dementia

It is sobering to realize that the first edition of this book did not require a section on AIDS-related dementia, AIDS dementia complex, or what is more accurately known as human immunodeficiency virus (HIV) dementia (or HIV organic mental disorder in the *Diagnostic and Statistical Manual of Mental Disorders* [*DSM-IV-R*; American Psychiatric Association, 2000]). Since publication of the first edition, AIDS and HIV infection have become even more serious public health problems, and researchers and clinicians have learned that HIV infection can result in a subcortical dementia. Interestingly, whereas the number of deaths in the United States secondary to AIDS has decreased since the second edition of this book, the number of individuals living with AIDS has increased. Highly active antiretroviral therapy has played an important part in the increased lifespan (Centers for Disease Control, 2001).

Early researchers dismissed the behavioral changes they observed in HIV-positive patients as sequelae of the emotional response to the disease, but it has been since demonstrated that neurological complications occur in about 40% of patients with AIDS, and in 10% of these patients, the neurological manifestations will constitute the first clinical signs of disease (Pajeau & Roman, 1992). In one study at The Johns Hopkins University, one patient in four presented with evidence of an AIDS dementia complex before any other clinical symptom was present (Dal Canto, 1989). Ho, Bredesen, Vinters, and Daar (1989) reported that 80–90% of the brains of AIDS patients they examined demonstrated neuropathological abnormalities. MRI studies have global and diffuse atrophy, isolated focal lesions, and subcortical hyperintensity.

It is important that HIV dementia be considered in the differential diagnosis of older patients suspected of having a dementia illness. This discrimination is often not easily made, and there is perhaps no other area in which there is so much overlap between psychiatric conditions (e.g., acute stress reactions, adjustment disorders, reactive psychoses, and depression) and neurological disease. At the very least, the clinician should search for risk factors for AIDS. If they are present, serological testing should be recommended (Maj, 1990).

Patients with HIV dementias present with cognitive, motor, and behavioral symptoms. The cognitive signs of HIV dementia include memory disturbance, lack of ability to concentrate, motor weakness, executive dysfunction, and confusion. The onset of these symptoms is insidious. Motor symptoms include loss of balance, clumsiness, and weakness in the lower extremities. Behavioral symptoms include apathy, blunted affect, social withdrawal, and loss of libido. Depression is a frequent complaint, and the psychomotor slowing observed in these patients resembles that found in clinical depression; however, when depression accompanies HIV dementia, it is resistant to treatment with medication.

On neurological examination, the patient with an HIV dementia will often exhibit gait ataxia and hyperreflexia. *Dysdiadochokinesis* (difficulty executing rapid alternating movements) is common. Other neurological symptoms, such as tremors, primitive reflexes, or myoclonus, may be present. Brain scans often show cortical atrophy, dilated ventricles, and white matter disease.

Neuropsychological evaluation of patients with HIV dementia remains the most sensitive measure for identifying the early and subtle changes associated with this disorder, and it provides far more sensitive data than that available from standardized MSEs (Pajeau & Roman, 1992). Although the difficulties documented by neuropsychological testing will be a function of the severity and stage of the disorder, it is common to find that patients with HIV dementia have difficulty with tasks requiring complex sequencing, fine rapid motor movement, processing speed, and visual scanning (Redmond & Wilson, 1990). An analysis of HIV-infected patients who were asymptomatic indicated that subtle cognitive impairment occurs (Heaton et al., 1995).

Butters et al. (1990) have proposed an extended (7–9 hours) and a brief (1–2 hours) neuropsychological battery for assessing the cognitive changes that occur in HIV seropositive, asymptomatic individuals. This includes typical areas of cognitive assessment, such as attention, processing speed, working memory, visual–spatial and constructional abilities, language, abstract reasoning, motor speed, and psychiatric symptoms. The tests associated with these cognitive areas are described in subsequent chapters of the book.

Although HIV dementias result in cortical changes (e.g., cerebral atrophy), they are generally regarded, along with Huntington's and Parkinson's diseases, as *subcortical dementias* because of the salience of the white matter changes that occur with the disease (Navia, Jordan, & Price, 1986). In general, cortical dementias result in specific deficits such as aphasia, agnosia, amnesia, and acalculia. Subcortical dementias spare language, but result in dysarthria, abnormal posture and gait, bradykinesia, and movement disorders such as chorea, rigidity, ataxia, and tremor (Kaemingk & Kaszniak, 1989).

As mentioned previously, highly active antiretroviral therapy has assisted in decreasing AIDS-related mortality. Interestingly, this treatment has also been found to stabilize brain abnormalities that are found on MRIs (Stankoff et al., 2001) and decrease neurocognitive decline (Maschke et al., 2000). Psychomotor and motor speed seems to improve with treatment. However, subtle cognitive impairment exists (see Sacktor, 2002 for review).

HEAD TRAUMA

Each year, approximately 1.3 million people are treated for head trauma in hospital emergency departments, with many more not seeking medical attention (Jager, Weiss, Cohen, & Pepe, 2000). It is an area of critical importance in neuropsychology, because detailed psychometric assessment will frequently reveal deficits in the head-injured patient when all other neurodiagnostic tests are negative. The psychologist must be sensitive to the medical sequelae that can result from trauma, and must appreciate the physics of head trauma, as well as have a basic understanding of the structure of the brain and skull, to approach the head-injured patient with any real understanding of the nature of the injury. In addition, the general clinician must be sensitive to possible untoward developments, such as cerebrospinal rhinorrhea (leakage of CSF from the nose secondary to a traumatic fracture of the cribriform plate), which may signal the need for immediate medical referral, because CSF leakage provides an easy route for subsequent brain infection.

Traumatic head injuries are traditionally classified as concussions, contusions, or open-head injuries. The concussion occurs when the brain is jarred. Strub and Black (1988) define a concussion as "an acute impairment of cerebral function secondary to an impact injury to the head in which the following are usually, but not invariably, present: amnesia, loss of consciousness, and complete recovery" (p. 316). The amnesia can be either retrograde (for events prior to the moment of injury) or anterograde (for events that occurred subsequent to the injury); neither type of amnesia necessarily predicts permanent brain injury. However, with *repeated* concussions, permanent damage is likely to occur. This chronic condition is referred to as traumatic encephalopathy. It is also known as dementia pugilistica or punch-drunk syndrome, because of its frequent occurrence in boxers. The syndrome is clearly evident in many aging boxers and includes dysarthric speech, slowness of thought, emotional lability, mild paranoia, and difficulty with impulse control. A good illustration of dementia pugilistica is available in the Martin Scorsese film *Raging Bull*.

A more common result of even a single concussion is the controversial postconcussion syndrome, characterized by problems with memory, impaired concentration, headaches, intellectual and physical fatigue, anxiety, dizziness, and increased sensitivity to noise. Impotence and irritability are also frequently noted following concussions. Whereas persistent postconcussive syndrome has clearly been identified, there is often a concern that a patient is feigning symptoms for either monetary or other reasons. This consideration is further discussed in chapter 11.

Contusions are more serious traumatic injuries in which the brain is actually bruised, typically from its impact with the skull. The contusion can result either from direct bleeding at the site of impact or from the tearing of adjacent blood vessels connecting the brain and meninges. The behavioral effects of the contusion last longer than those of the concussion, and the neuropsychological findings tend to be more focal. Basal frontotemporal contusions occur most frequently. The contusion can produce a *coup* injury at the point of impact; this is most common when a moving object (e.g., a blackjack) hits a stationary head. *Contrecoup* injuries occur when a moving head hits a stationary object (e.g., when a head hits a steering wheel during a motor vehicle accident); these injuries are characterized by damage to tissue opposite the site of impact, and occur with most cases of posterior head injuries that produce marked frontal and anterior temporal lobe damage in those areas in which the brain rebounds against the opposite end of the skull. In contrast, contrecoup injuries to the occipital lobes themselves are quite rare, probably because of the smooth contour of the occipital bones and the absence of bony projections on the inner side of the posterior skull (Reitan & Wolfson, 1985).

Open-head injuries and brain lacerations occur most often in wartime. They produce focal lesions, but the resulting edema and bleeding may result in diffuse damage with multiple behavioral deficits. Patients with open-head injuries typically make rapid progress, and the majority of those who survive their injuries return to work. If the injury severs a major cerebral artery, pronounced deficits and eventual death are the most likely outcomes.

Many head-injury patients will be comatose for days or weeks after their injuries. The duration of coma has been shown to correlate well with mortality, psychosocial dependency, and intellectual impairment, especially in patients over the age of 30 (Strub & Black, 1988).

The Glasgow Coma Scale provides a convenient and objective method for rating level of consciousness. The scale assesses three areas: eye opening, motor responding, and verbal responding. Each area is scored, and scores are summed; the summed scores can range from 3 to 15. A score of 15 indicates that the patient is alert and responsive; a score of 3 indicates a deep coma. Scores between 3 and 15 indicate various levels of alertness, eye-tracking skills, and ability to demonstrate appropriate motor responses. Patients with scores of 7 and below are considered to be comatose. The Glasgow Coma Scale is discussed in detail in chapter 5.

The total duration of posttraumatic amnesia is a more useful predictor of degree of injury and likelihood of recovery than either retrograde amnesia or the length of time a patient is comatose. It is also a significant predictor of the length of time before a patient can return to work.

Table 1.3

RELATIONSHIP BETWEEN POSTTRAUMATIC AMNESIA AND SEVERITY OF INJURY

POSTTRAUMATIC AMNESIA	CLASSIFICATION
< 1 hour	Mild
1–24 hours	Moderate
1–7 days	Severe
More than 7 days	Very severe

Table 1.3 lists the conventional nomenclature for rating the severity of head injuries. There is no completely agreed-upon severity index of closed-head injuries. Note that the duration of posttraumatic amnesia is measured from the time of the injury until the restoration of continuous awareness; islets of memory do not qualify as evidence of restoration of memory functioning.

Most closed-head injuries produce deficits that implicate both hemispheres. Motor and sensory deficits tend to be less pronounced than those that accompany vascular disorders. However, traumatic vascular injuries, such as epidural, subdural, subarachnoid, and intracerebral hemorrhages, are frequent concomitants of both open- and closed-head injuries. Injuries to the frontal lobes are common, resulting in loss of inhibition and behavioral control and impaired ability in simultaneous processing and in processing complex stimuli. Memory skills are frequently impaired. Traditional measures of global intellectual ability are frequently insensitive to the effects of head injuries, because the handicap that results from a head injury is not one of intelligence, but rather one of attention, memory, and a broad range of information-processing skills (Bond, 1986). Head-injured patients deserve to be assessed with measures at least as sensitive as those we discuss later in this book. If at all possible, they should receive a comprehensive neuropsychological workup.

SEIZURE DISORDERS

Epilepsy is not a disease in its own right, but rather a symptom complex characteristic of a variety of disorders that alter brain function. It can be defined as the recurrent paroxysmal uncontrolled discharge of cerebral neurons in such a way as to interfere with normal activity. Seizure activity is most often the consequence of head trauma: seizures develop in about 5% of closed-head injuries and in more than 30% of head injuries in which the dura has been penetrated (Lishman, 1978). A variety of other disorders can insult neural tissue, including birth trauma, infectious disorders such as meningitis, toxins including mercury, vascular changes, metabolic or nutritional disturbances such as electrolyte and water imbalance or vitamin deficiency, neoplasms, and degenerative diseases such as MS. The disorder is termed *idiopathic epilepsy* when no discernible cause is present for the seizures that occur.

The incidence of epilepsy is approximately 1–4% in the general population, with the occurrence decidedly higher in males. There are approximately two and a half million epileptics in the United States today, 20% of whom are not adequately controlled by medication.

Seventy-five percent of seizure disorders begin before the age of 20; 30% begin by the age of 4. Less than 2% of seizure disorders have their onset after the age of 50 (Trauner, 1982). Onset of seizures in a patient after the age of 35 without clear causation must always lead to the presumptive diagnosis of a brain lesion, and these patients require immediate neurological evaluation.

A number of environmental stimuli may precipitate seizures in the susceptible individual. These include hyperventilation, sleep deprivation, sensory stimuli, trauma, hormonal changes, fever, emotional stress, and drugs (Pincus & Tucker, 1985).

Classification of seizure activity has always been somewhat arbitrary, imprecise, and sometimes confusing. However, the International Classification of Epileptic Seizures (Engel, 2001) has been widely accepted. This classification schema is reproduced in Table 1.4.

Partial seizures are so named because seizure activity begins locally, and only part of the brain is involved. Partial seizures with elementary symptoms involve focal motor or sensory symptoms (such as a twitching finger), which may escalate along one side of the body (a "Jacksonian march"), but which by definition never come to involve the entire brain and body. The motor disturbance usually begins distally and moves in a proximal direction, and the patient remains conscious throughout the event.

Partial seizures with complex symptoms are of particular interest to the psychologist. These seizures have traditionally been called psychomotor seizures, or sometimes temporal lobe seizures (somewhat

Table 1.4

OUTLINE OF THE INTERNATIONAL CLASSIFICATION OF EPILEPSY

I. Partial seizures (seizures beginning locally)
   A. With elementary symptomatology (generally without impairment of consciousness)
      1. With motor symptoms
      2. With special sensory or somatosensory symptoms
      3. With autonomic symptoms
      4. Compound forms
   B. With complex symptomatology (generally with some impairment of consciousness)
      1. With impairment of consciousness only
      2. With cognitive symptomatology
      3. With affective symptomatology
      4. With pseudosensory symptomatology
      5. With psychomotor symptomatology (automatisms)
      6. Compound forms
   C. Partial seizures, secondarily generalized
II. Generalized seizures (bilaterally symmetrical without known local onset with loss of consciousness)
   A. Absence
   B. Tonic/clonic
   C. Tonic
   D. Clonic
   E. Bilateral epileptic myoclonus
   F. Atonic
   G. Akinetic
   H. Infantile spasms
   I. Myoclonic
III. Unilateral seizures
IV. Unclassified seizures

incorrectly, because they can also originate in the inferior medial aspects of the frontal lobe). This is the most common form of seizure, and its first occurrence is typically around the age of puberty. Although the origin is focal, these lesions result in symptoms that are complex and varied. There is a prodromal period that may be characterized by feelings of impending disaster. During the ictal event itself, the patient experiences an altered state of awareness and may hallucinate. Feelings of *déjà vu* (in which new experiences seem familiar) and *jamais vu* (in which familiar settings or situations seem unusual and unreal) are common. Oral or facial automatisms such as blinking, smacking, and chewing are often present. While seizing, the patient will move about and may interact with other people in his environment; however, *the person having partial complex seizures will not engage in structured, purposeful, and sequential activity.* (Jack Ruby's lawyers argued that he was experiencing a psychomotor seizure when he shot Lee Harvey Oswald. However, it is unlikely that a seizure patient would be able to carry out the complex chain of events required to complete an assassination successfully. In general, the incidence of violent behavior in psychomotor seizures is quite low.) After a seizure, the patient is typically confused and depressed, and there is a total amnesia for the events of the ictal period.

Hallucinations are rare in simple partial seizures, but common in partial complex seizures, especially with seizure foci in the posterior part of the temporal lobe (Oxbury & Duchowney, 2000). Visual hallucinations are the most common (18%), followed by auditory (16%), olfactory (12%), and gustatory (3%) hallucinations. Rage reactions occur in about 2% of cases, whereas the sensation of déjà vu occurs in 14% of seizures. Visual hallucinations originating in the temporal lobe tend to be complex and detailed, whereas those that originate in the occipital area are simpler, and appear as colored lines, stars, and circles in the contralateral visual field. When auditory hallucinations occur with partial complex seizures, they are usually unformed and the contents are rarely bizarre, threatening, or condemning (Kilpatrick & Hall, 1980).

There has been a great deal of interest in the "temporal lobe personality," which is believed to be associated with partial complex seizures. Patients with complex partial seizures often exhibit emotional lability, sudden outbursts of anger, circumstantiality, and decreased frustration tolerance. They are also noted to be hyperreligious, hyposexual, viscous, and hypergraphic. Hyposexuality results from loss of interest rather than from loss of ability. These patients also become quite serious about even minor matters and develop a fascination with details and minutia. Psychic symptoms may include changes in speech, language, or memory (Browne & Holmes, 2004).

Generalized seizures are bilaterally symmetrical and involve both hemispheres of the brain. Their origin is deep in the brain, and these seizures result in loss of consciousness. In *absence* (petit mal) seizures, there is a brief (5–15-second) loss of consciousness without loss of muscle tone. The seizure is accompanied by a vacant stare and occasional eye blinking. The EEG almost always shows 3-second wave and pike discharges during the ictal event. The disorder occurs almost exclusively in young children, who may have multiple episodes each day. The diagnosis should be questioned if the phenomenon occurs fewer than five times per day (Lishman, 1978). The disorder is *not* associated with diminished intelligence, and the condition almost always clears after puberty.

Generalized tonic–clonic seizures (grand mal seizures) involve a sudden loss of consciousness with tonic rigidity followed by clonic jerking. The ictal event lasts for 1–2 minutes and may involve loss of consciousness, tongue biting, and urinary and fecal incontinence. Following the seizure, there is a period of postictal confusion accompanied by headache and fatigue, along with a total amnesia for the ictal event. Contrary to popular lore, nothing should be inserted in the mouth of the patient during the seizure episode; instead, the head should be protected and emotional support should be provided when the seizure ends.

Although the EEG will almost always be abnormal during an actual ictal event, the simple waking EEG will be normal in at least 50% of bona fide seizure patients. Greater accuracy occurs when sleep deprivation, photic stimulation, or hyperventilation studies are used. A left-hemisphere EEG focus predicts diminished verbal IQ (relative to performance IQ scores), whereas the reverse is true with patients with a right-hemisphere focus (lower performance IQ relative to verbal abilities). In general, the severity of neuropsychological impairment correlates well with longer duration and earlier onset of seizures. Neuropsychological impairment also correlates with seizure frequency, and tonic–clonic seizures are associated with a greater degree of neuropsychological deficits than complex partial seizures (Reitan & Wolfson, 1985).

CONCLUSIONS

Cognitive deficits almost routinely accompany compromised neurological functioning. Although these deficits may be readily apparent at times, often subtle changes or impairments exist. An astute clinician needs to be aware of the neurodiagnostic possibilities for behavioral and cognitive alterations in functioning. Although technology has improved our ability to diagnose and treat these conditions, the behavioral and cognitive changes that occur are often the first indication of a brain-based disorder. Early recognition of these symptoms can improve long-term outcome. It is, therefore, important for clinicians to be aware of the behavioral and cognitive tendencies of different neurological disorders.

2 Psychiatric Disorders With Neurological Implications

The distinction between neurological and psychiatric disorders is a false dichotomy, and the clinician must be aware of organic correlates, genetic involvement, cognitive impairment, and environmental factors in every patient evaluated. However, for the sake of tradition and convenience, we follow the practice of separating neurological and psychiatric disorders. In this chapter, we briefly discuss the neuropsychological relevance of a variety of disorders traditionally viewed as functional. These include schizophrenia, affective illness, anxiety disorders, attention deficit disorder, and, to a lesser extent alcoholism. There has been a plethora of studies examining these areas over the past 2 decades. For the sake of space, each disorder will be briefly discussed.

SCHIZOPHRENIA

Professionals working in the mental health field have been trained to recognize schizophrenia. It is a common disorder with a worldwide incidence of at least 1%, and one cannot work for long in the mental health system without encountering patients diagnosed with schizophrenia. However, perhaps because of its relative frequency, it is easy to overdiagnose schizophrenia, particularly in the African American community (Bresnahan et al., 2007; Strakowski, McElroy, Keck, & West, 1996).

Schizophrenia is easier to recognize than define. Bleuler originally described the disorder in terms of four fundamental symptoms. He said the schizophrenic patient displayed defects in *association* and *affect*, and was characterized by *ambivalence* and *autism*. Although conceptually neat and alluringly alliterative, there are a number of practical problems with Bleuler's criteria. Most important, Bleuler's symptoms lack precision. Schneider improved the situation somewhat by developing first-rank and second-rank criteria for the diagnosis of schizophrenia. Schneiderian first-rank symptoms include auditory hallucinations, delusional experiences, and distorted perceptions. Secondary symptoms include blocking, concrete thinking, and distorted ideas of reference. Pincus and Tucker (1985) listed six major criteria for the diagnosis of schizophrenia: (a) a thought disorder characterized by either hallucinations of delusions in the absence of some known cause, or some other form of conceptual disorganization; (b) early onset of symptoms; (c) absence of major affective symptoms; (d) absence of major neurological deficits; (e) a progressively deteriorating course or an intermittent course with remissions, and (f) a history of schizophrenia in close relatives (that contributes to, but is not necessary for, the diagnosis). The *Diagnostic and Statistical Manual of Mental Health Disorders* (*DSM-IV-TR*; American Psychiatric Association, 2000) criteria include the presence of at least two of five specific signs (e.g., delusions, hallucinations, disorganized speech), deterioration from a previous higher level of functioning, and continuous signs of the illness for at least six months at some time in the patient's life. In addition, it is necessary to rule out schizoaffective and mood disorders, as well as substance disorders and general medical conditions that might account for the patient's symptoms. Psychological tests are specifically helpful in meeting this last criterion; however, *the diagnosis of schizophrenia is frequently made without consideration of the plethora of neurological disorders that can present with schizophrenia-like symptoms*. For example, unsuspected structural lesions are found in the brains of 5–10% of chronic psychiatric patients, and meningiomas are found twice as often in psychiatric patients as in the general population (Lechtenberg, 1982). Many of the signs of schizophrenia (e.g., poverty of content, word salad, blunted affect) are found with specific neurological diseases, and the effects of a lesion may mimic a schizophrenic process. We cannot emphasize strongly enough that patients suspected of being schizophrenic should receive neuropsychological screening to test for specific cortical deficits that may exist in addition to the more diffuse signs of schizophrenia. If specific neuropsychological deficits exist, medical referral is warranted.

Favorable prognostic signs in schizophrenia include sudden onset of the disorder, the presence of conspicuous precipitating factors, the presence of anxiety or affective symptoms, family history of affective illness, a history of good social adjustment, marriage, employment, medication compliance, and cooperation by the patient. Significant negative predictors include onset of the disorder in childhood or puberty and a family history of schizophrenia. Further, it is thought that approximately 75% of patients diagnosed with schizophrenia have significant cognitive impairment. Widespread neuropsychological impairment has been reported, including attention, memory, executive functioning, motor skills, and intelligence. Cognitive impairment is also thought to be related to functional outcome.

Although *DSM-IV-TR* classifies schizophrenia into specific subtypes (disorganized, catatonic, paranoid, undifferentiated, and residual types), we find it more useful simply to classify patients as being process or reactive schizophrenics. This dichotomy has been used by clinicians for years in one form or another. Process schizophrenia is characterized by gradual onset of illness, social isolation and withdrawal, and poor prognosis. Impaired performance on neuropsychological tests is almost always present. Computed tomography (CT) or magnetic resonance imaging (MRI) scans often reveal structural brain deficits, and neurological soft signs are common. In contrast, reactive schizophrenia is characterized by rapid onset and a better prognosis. Neuropsychological deficits are less likely to be present, and specific neurological anomalies are rare. There are fewer soft neurological signs on examination, and there is typically a better response to medication. Reactive schizophrenics are characterized by positive symptoms (delusions, hallucinations, and thought disorder), whereas process schizophrenics are found to have primarily negative symptoms (flat affect, little motivation, poverty of thought and speech). Crow (1982) characterizes these as Type I (reactive) or Type II (process) syndromes. *Although specific neurological deficits may be found in either group, evidence of brain impairment is far more likely to be found in those patients with primarily negative symptoms.*

Neuropsychological assessment of psychiatric patients, particularly process/chronic schizophrenics, has almost always yielded a high number of what have traditionally been assumed to be "false-positive" diagnoses, as these patients perform in a manner similar to patients with demonstrable brain pathology (tumors, dementias, strokes, etc.). This finding, along with the increased incidence of neurological soft signs (e.g., electroencephalograph [EEG] abnormalities), led some investigators to hypothesize that a sizable number of schizophrenics did, in fact, have specific brain impairment. Imaging studies have supported this hypothesis. Compared with normal controls, schizophrenics have larger cerebral ventricles, increased sulcal widths, increased width of the interhemispheric fissure, cerebellar atrophy, and a reversal of typical patterns of asymmetry (i.e., wider left frontal and right occipital lobes relative to normal controls). They also show decreased tissue density in the left hemisphere and an overall brain volume decrease. These differences do not correlate with age, length of hospitalization, or medication use. Patients who demonstrate the greatest structural deficits tend to perform most poorly on neuropsychological tests (Wedding, 1986). Although some authors have argued that the anterior and dorsolateral portions of the frontal lobes are dysfunctional in schizophrenics and the left hemisphere is more affected by the disease process than the right hemisphere (Henn & Nasrallah, 1982; Nasrallah & Weinberger, 1986), others have demonstrated a temporal lobe, basal ganglia, and either the right or left hemisphere involvement (Blanchard & Neale, 1994). These inconsistencies are likely due to the wide heterogeneity of the disorder. Regardless, schizophrenia research has come full circle, and we are once again at the point of trying to understand the neurobiology of *dementia praecox*.

Findings such as these illustrate the futility of attempting to find neuropsychological measures to classify patients into two arbitrary groups: psychiatric (functional) or neurological (organic). The dichotomy is artificial, and substantial overlap exists between the two populations. It is often more useful to describe the nature of the thought disorder that occurs in the schizophrenic patient and to screen for signs of specific focal damage that may point to remediable disorders (e.g., shunting in the case of normal pressure hydrocephalus).

Schizophrenia-like episodes have been associated with trauma, neoplasms, encephalitis, degenerative disease, autoimmune diseases, vascular disorders, and cerebral anoxia. However, Pincus and Tucker (1985) point out that disorientation, memory deficits, confusion, and fluctuating states of consciousness are more commonly encountered with specific neurological disease than with schizophrenia. In addition, acute neurological disorders are typically characterized by: (a) a good premorbid social history; (b) abrupt changes in personality, mood, or ability; (c) rapid fluctuations in mental status; and (d) a lack of response to either psychotherapeutic or pharmacological intervention efforts.

Complex partial seizures can sometimes mimic schizophrenia, especially when there is a left-sided anterior temporal focus (Flor-Henry, 1976). However, the absence of precipitating events, the shorter duration of bizarre behavior, the presence of an aura, and postictal drowsiness should help identify the recurrent complex partial seizure disorder.

AFFECTIVE DISORDERS

Affective disorders are the most common psychiatric conditions treated in America today; they are also the disorders most commonly misdiagnosed as dementias. Because of the ubiquitous nature of this problem, it is essential that the clinician be sensitive to the possibility that a major depression is present in the patient who presents with cognitive failure, because *affective illness frequently mimics primary degenerative dementia, especially in the elderly*. In addition, many medical conditions present with depression as a primary initial symptom: these examples include anemia, multiple sclerosis, Cushing's disease, thyroid and parathyroid disease, acromegaly, systemic lupus erythematosus, and ulcerative colitis (Hall, 1980). In addition, heart disease and cancer can initially present with the symptoms of fatigue and depression.

The problem of diagnosis is complicated by the fact that although depression can mimic organic mental syndromes, it can also be a part of the presenting picture of true brain disease. For example, it is estimated that approximately 50% of individuals with dementia have depression at some point of their illness. Depression is also common with the catastrophic reaction that sometimes accompanies left-hemisphere lesions.

The differential diagnosis of dementia and depression is one of a neuropsychologist's most challenging (and most common) referral questions. It is a situation in which *good performance is more helpful than poor performance: good performance can help rule out brain disease, whereas poor performance does little to rule in the diagnosis of organic mental disease.*

Although poor test performance is characteristic of the patient with a major affective illness, some general principles can help the clinician make a more positive diagnosis. For example, in the depressed patient, it is common for complaints and concerns about failing memory to be worse than objective performance on memory examinations. *Poor performance on tests of immediate memory and attention only should alert the clinician to the possibility of depression.* In addition, the psychologist often finds that verbal tasks are more helpful than nonverbal tests, because depressed people typically perform quite poorly on those nonverbal tests that require motoric responding. This is likely due to slowed processing speed and decreased cognitive efficiency. Poor performance on motor tasks is especially common when the test is timed. (Construction tasks are a possible exception. Given sufficient time, most depressed patients can adequately reproduce simple geometric forms, whereas the demented patient may have a great deal of difficulty.) Across a variety of tests, depressed patients tend to display deficits suggestive of frontotemporal deficits.

The psychologist should be especially sensitive to the likelihood of pseudodementia when performance on a screening battery is inconsistent from test to test, especially when similar abilities are being assessed by two separate tests. "I don't know" responses and paucity of effort are common in depression, but with encouragement, the patient will often respond correctly. However, it may be difficult for the truly depressed patient to maintain a consistently acceptable level of energy and effort, especially on timed visual motor integration tasks. We have also found it helpful to administer the Controlled Word Association Test (discussed later in this book) to patients we suspect of having pseudodementia. Not surprisingly, a content analysis frequently reveals the presence of numerous responses suggestive of hopelessness and helplessness. Patient affect also may be diagnostically important. Although facial immobility of the depressed patient will sometimes resemble that of the patient with Parkinson's disease, more commonly, one finds depressed affect that may prove helpful in differential diagnosis. Any family history of affective illness or suicide, as well as any past personal history of mood swings or manic episodes, may be diagnostically important, as well.

Other dimensions separate the demented patient from the patient with a pseudodementia. There is more commonly some precipitating event (e.g., retirement or the death of a spouse) in depression, and the depressed patient is less likely to try to hide mistakes or to make excuses for poor performance on psychological testing. A history of marked guilt (occurring *before* the development of impaired cognition) suggests depressive pseudodementia. Associated vegetative signs of depression (e.g., weight loss, early morning awakenings) can occur with organic mental syndromes, but are more common with depression. Progressive deterioration of functioning on serial testing would be more likely to occur in the patient with true brain disease, and a simple "Spike Two" profile would be somewhat less likely on a Minnesota Multiphasic Personality Inventory (MMPI-II; Butcher, Dahlstrom, Graham, Tellegen, & Kaemmer, 1989) taken by a patient with an organic illness.

There are other differences between the patient with true dementia and the patient with pseudodementia. With true dementia, onset of symptoms is more likely to be insidious, with a gradual course; with pseudodementias, the onset is more acute and the course more rapid. The demented patient often finds that his or her symptoms are exacerbated in the evening (sundowning); the depressed patient is likely to complain that his or her problems are worse in the morning. Adamant refusal to cooperate with testing is more common in the demented patient, whereas the depressed individual is more likely to cooperate superficially, but put forth little effort on the actual tests that are administered. Finally, in the early stages of a dementia illness, social skills are likely to be well preserved, whereas they will be clearly impaired in the patient with a pseudodementia.

The neurophysiology and cognitive abilities in patients diagnosed with bipolar disorder have been extensively examined during the past 2 decades. Although older studies suggested that bipolar disorder is primarily due to a right-hemisphere dysfunction, neuroimaging research indicates that it is predominantly due to an anterior limbic network dysfunction (Strakowski, DelBello, & Adler, 2005). Cognitive impairment is also typically found in these patients, even during periods of euthymia. However, some performance on various cognitive measures, including memory, attention, and processing speed, may be variable, dependent on mood state.

ANXIETY DISORDERS

There are a wide variety of anxiety disorders, each of which has different neurophysiological and neurocognitive abnormalities. For example, although imaging studies indicate a prefrontal-limbic dysfunction in patients with generalized anxiety disorder (GAD), cognitive performance on tests can be inconsistent, due to the variability in the patient's ability to cope with his/her anxiety about completing the tests. Further, there is only a modest genetic component to GAD. In comparison, patients with panic disorder are found to have a dysregulation of the cingulate system. Panic disorder is thought to have a high genetic involvement, with molecular genetic testing indicating involvement in chromosomes 15 and 7q.

Obsessive-compulsive disorder (OCD) is another example of the clear neurological involvement in psychiatric illness. Up to 60% of patients with OCD have a first-degree relative with OCD. Genetic tests have demonstrated abnormalities in chromosome 9q. The basal ganglia is clearly involved in the expression of OCD, as evidenced by the fact that damage to that brain region leads to OCD behaviors in animals (Smolinsky et al., 2009). Further, individuals with OCD have poor performance on measures examining cognitive flexibility and selective attention.

Given the high occurrence of trauma-related events in our society, posttraumatic stress disorder (PTSD) has increasingly been studied from a neurobiological perspective. Imaging results indicate that PTSD is associated with decreased hippocampal volume, dysregulation of the hypothalamic–pituitary–adrenal (HPA) axis, and neuroadrenergic activation. Elevated PTSD symptoms are significantly associated with executive dysfunction (Leskin & White, 2007). PTSD with prolonged traumatic cognitions can also result in difficulties occurring in attention, learning, fluency, memory, and working memory deficits (Galletly, Clark, McFarlane, & Weber, 2001; Uddo, Vasterling, Brailey, & Sutker, 1993; Yehuda et al., 1995).

ATTENTION-DEFICIT/HYPERACTIVITY DISORDERS

Once thought to be exclusively a childhood-related disorder, attention-deficit/ hyperactivity disorder (ADHD) appears to persist into adulthood for many patients. The American Psychological Association even recognized that ADHD persists into adulthood in the *DSM-IV* (APA, 1994). Whereas the clinical characteristics of childhood ADHD include inattention, hyperactivity, impulsivity, and executive dysfunction, typically, executive dysfunction is the prominent feature in adult ADHD (Biederman, Mick, & Faraone, 2000). Executive dysfunction, also discussed in a later chapter, is used to describe higher-order cognitive skills, such as organization, inhibition, planning, and motivation. Consistent with these findings are imaging studies that have indicated involvement in the prefrontal system, as well as possibly the striatum (Diamond, 2007; Spencer, Biederman, Wilens, & Faraone, 2002). Genetic studies have found dopaminergic system involvement, as well (Swanson et al., 2000).

ALCOHOLISM

The practicing psychologist will frequently see patients whose cognitive functions have been adversely affected by substance abuse. It is critical that the clinician be sensitive to the effects of alcohol on brain function, because *cognitive impairment and cerebral atrophy will appear long before significant liver damage or other overt medical signs of alcoholism.* Psychological screening for cerebral impairment and memory dysfunction may be especially important in these patients, because social and verbal skills are relatively preserved, and the existence of brain dysfunction may not be readily apparent on medical examination or on a casual mental-status examination.

Korsakoff's psychosis is the brain syndrome most clearly associated with chronic alcoholism. This disorder is characterized by impairment of recent memory that is markedly greater than other cognitive deficiencies. Remote memory is also impaired, but to a less striking degree. These memory deficits are actually secondary to nutritional inadequacy, and result from shortages of thiamine in the diet of the alcoholic that contribute to degeneration of the cortical mantel and atrophy of the thalamus and mammillary bodies.

Patients with Korsakoff's disease present with flattened affect, and typically have little insight. They are likely to deny both the severity of their alcohol abuse and the significance of their memory failure. Immediate memory, as measured on tests such as Digit Span, tends to be intact, and often relatively good performance is present on most intelligence measures. However, there will typically be at least a 20-point discrepancy between full-scale IQ and the memory performance, Marked deficits will be present on any sort of delayed memory task, and confabulation may be present. *However, contrary to popular clinical lore, confabulation is neither consistently present, nor is it a requirement for the diagnosis* (Adams & Victor, 1977). The personality changes associated with Korsakoff's disease most often involve passivity and apathy.

Although the diagnosis of Korsakoff's disease highlights the presence of memory impairment, the condition almost always accompanies *Wernicke's disease*, a disorder characterized by the triad of mental confusion, gait ataxia, and ocular abnormalities. The patient with Wernicke's disease is characterized by a wide-based stance and a slow and uncertain gait. Ocular abnormalities include ophthalmoplegias (weakness or paralysis of conjugate gaze) and nystagmus. The confusional state tends to be global, with the specific impairment of memory alluded to previously. Because these memory deficits are virtually always present, many authors refer to this condition as Wernicke–Korsakoff's syndrome.

CONCLUSIONS

Space limitations preclude a more detailed discussion of the full range of psychopathology likely to be encountered by the clinician. The varieties and vicissitudes of mental illness and brain disease are such that a primer of this sort can only highlight the most common problems that occur. However, research has consistently demonstrated that psychiatric illness is associated with cognitive difficulties. Although the cognitive problems are varied, efforts are being made to understand which cognitive areas are impaired for various disorders. These cognitive areas will be discussed in the following chapters.

3 Approaches to Neurological Assessment

A neurologist is a physician who specializes in disorders of the nervous system. Neurologists see patients who have a wide variety of disorders such as closed-head injury, seizure disorders, dementing disorders, including Alzheimer's, Parkinson's, or Huntington's, and the various cerebral palsy conditions. Neurologists also see patients on the basis of their symptoms, rather than their diagnoses. These include patients with headaches or chronic medical pain, or patients with memory complaints or muscular disorders.

Most of the patients seen by a neurologist have been referred by other health care professionals who have performed their own assessments. Recent advances in medical science have produced new laboratory tests for the neurologist, including imaging (computed tomography [CT], magnetic resonance imaging [MRI], single-photon emission computerized tomography [SPECT]), electrical tests (electroencephalograph [EEG], electromyograph [EMG]), and even genetic tests. However, neurology as a practice is still defined by the careful history. Frequently, the neurologist will perform a comprehensive physical examination prior to the neurological examination. Although the physical exam conducted by a neurologist is similar to typical exams performed by other physicians, the neurological evaluation is different from that which would be conducted by most other health care professionals. The neurological evaluation concentrates on an assessment of nervous system functions. All areas of nervous system function are likely to be screened, and more in-depth assessments are reserved for those areas that have been identified as problematic, either in the history or in the referral. Despite the heterogeneity of neurological evaluations, they are all likely to be organized around certain areas of nervous system functioning. The neurologist will generally test the functioning of the cranial nerves, the cerebellum, the motor system, the sensory system, the reflexes, and the cerebral functions. The following descriptions are cursory, and are only intended to inform the general clinician of the procedures that are likely to occur after the patient is referred to a neurologist.

The neurologist uses tests in a somewhat different way from the psychologist, who associates the word "test" with a set of procedures that have rigidly standardized administration and scoring procedures. In the psychological test, measurement results in a numerical score that is interpreted via reference to a set of normative data. With the exception of lab tests, for the neurologist, a test is a set of procedures that are more loosely standardized than for psychologists. It is a challenge of a function, and the result is frequently binary—absence or presence of impairment. There is more improvisation occurring in a neurological examination than in a psychological test.

As noted previously, the information derived from a neurological test is usually dichotomous. For example, in testing the reflexes, a set of fairly standardized procedures may be used to elicit the reflex. The information derived is whether or not the reflex occurred following the eliciting stimulus. Sometimes this information is qualified by an indication of whether the reflex was normal, exaggerated, or minimal. However, in contrast to the psychological test, scoring the neurological test is by comparison with a set of informal, internal norms. The neurologist decides whether the reflex is normal by comparing it with other reflexes that she has seen. The experience and observation acumen of the neurologist are of paramount importance in the diagnostic process.

THE NEUROLOGICAL EVALUATION

The outpatient neurological evaluation begins when the patient walks in the door. The inpatient evaluation begins when the physician walks in the hospital room. The neurologist will pay attention to numerous aspects of the patient's behavior throughout the evaluation. During the initial interview, the neurologist will note the hygiene, grooming, and general appearance of the patient. The neurologist will also note the ability of the patient to use language, and use this information to formulate the later assessment of language functions.

Arousal

The neurologist will assess the level of arousal of the patient, sometimes using one of the methods discussed in the section on arousal in the chapter of this book dealing with the mental status examination (MSE), and sometimes using a more informal method. If the patient appears to be unresponsive to verbal stimulation, the neurologist may evaluate the responsiveness of the patient to tactile stimulation, including responsiveness to painful stimulation. The level of alertness is noted, and a subjective narrative of the level is usually stated in the report.

History

The next step in the neurological examination is usually to take a detailed history. Because the neurologist is more interested than the general clinician in certain aspects of the history, the neurological history is likely to go into more depth in those areas. The neurologist will also perform an MSE similar to the MSE described in this book. However, the MSE given by the neurologist is less likely to make use of psychological tests, and is more likely to use informal procedures for the assessment of mental status. If there is a suspicion that the individual is exhibiting cognitive impairment, or if there is a question as to the etiology of the observed cognitive difficulties, the neurologist may refer to a neuropsychologist for a more in-depth assessment of cognitive processes.

Movement and Posture

The neurologist will next examine the station and gait of the patient. Station, or posture, is evaluated when the patient walks into the room, while the patient is sitting during the interview, and while the patient is performing those tasks suggested by the neurologist. Consistent leaning to one side is noted, as is the level of muscle tone in relaxed and active states. Sometimes the Romberg test is used. In this procedure, the patient is asked to stand with his feet side by side and touching each other. The ability of the patient to maintain an even posture and to remain erect without swaying is evaluated. If the individual being tested sways with eyes closed, but can stand with minimal swaying with eyes open, the test is said to be positive. The essence of the test is based on the fact that balance uses three symptoms of input: visual, proprioceptive, and vestibular. When the visual input is removed, difficulty maintaining balance can be due to either vestibular or proprioceptive dysfunction. Sometimes the patient will also be asked to stand on one foot to evaluate the same processes. The patient may also be asked to walk in a straight line, first freely and then heel to toe. A more difficult task requires the patient to hop on one leg for a short period. In all of these procedures, the strength, accuracy, speed, coordination, symmetry, and completeness of movement are assessed.

Cranial Nerves

An essential component of the neurological evaluation is the examination of the cranial nerves. The cranial nerves are a set of 12 pairs of nerves that connect the central nervous system (CNS) processors with the rest of the body. The olfactory cranial nerve (I) is evaluated by providing the patient with odiferous substances, separately to each nostril, and asking the patient to identify the substance. Substances used include soap, coffee, wintergreen, camphor, or tobacco. (Because damage to the first cranial nerve is rare, this portion of the evaluation of cranial nerves is sometimes omitted.)

The optic nerve (II) is examined by testing visual acuity and visual fields. These tests are informal, and may be followed up by more extensive testing procedures if the clinician deems it to be necessary. The oculomotor nerve (III) is assessed by examining for ptosis, appropriate dilation in response to light, and both the standing gaze and the ability of the eyes to follow a visual stimulus as it moves across the field of vision. The trochlear nerve (IV) is also assessed by examining the ability of the patient to track a stimulus. If the patient is unable to look downward and laterally, then the trochlear nerve is most likely affected. If the patient is unable to look laterally in one eye, then the respective abducens nerve (VI) is suspected of pathology. These symptoms are usually associated with complaints of diplopia. During this part of the evaluation, the neurologist is also examining for the presence of nystagmus. Cranial nerves III, IV, and VI are usually tested together.

The trigeminal cranial nerve (V) has a variety of functions that are assessed. Sensation for touch, pinpricks, heat, and cold is evaluated on both sides of the face while the patient's eyes are closed. By touching the cornea of the patient with a cotton swab, the neurologist can assess the corneal reflex. The neurologist will also ask the patient to close his jaws tightly, and then the neurologist will palpate the patient's jaw muscles in this part of the neurological examination. Finally, the maxillary reflex is tested by tapping the middle of the patient's chin when the mouth is slightly open.

The facial nerve (VII) is tested by examining the ability of the patient to imitate movements such as wrinkling the forehead, frowning, and raising the eyebrows. The patient is asked to tightly close his eyelids, and the neurologist will attempt to open the eyelids with his hand. The sense of taste, which is also associated with the VII cranial nerve, is assessed by placing salt and sugar on the anterior portion of the tongue.

The assessment of the acoustic nerve (VIII) has two major areas of evaluation that reflect its double set of functions. The tests of the vestibular functions of the VIII cranial nerve involve rotation and caloric tests requiring specialized equipment and complex procedures, and are, therefore, not usually included in the routine evaluation. The cochlear functions of the VIII cranial nerve are more amenable to clinical examination. The patient is asked to close one ear with a hand and the ability of the patient to detect the sound of a ticking watch at 3–4 feet is assessed. The sensitivity of the patient to vibrations from a tuning fork is assessed as the fork is held near each ear, as well as when the fork is in contact with the mastoid and the vertex of the skull. In addition, audiometric testing is sometimes used.

The glossopharyngeal nerve (IX) is tested by touching the posterior wall of the pharynx with a tongue depressor, which should result in contraction of the pharyngeal muscle. The results of this part of the evaluation are interpreted with reference to the results of the assessment of the vagus, because it is possible that the pharynx is innervated by the vagus in some patients. When this is true, the contraction of the pharyngeal muscles will be accompanied by a gag reflex.

The vagus nerve (X) is assessed by examining the palate, larynx, and pharynx. The patient is asked to perform simple verbalizations (the proverbial "Ah") while these muscle groups are examined. The patient is also asked to swallow.

The accessory nerve (XI) is assessed by having the patient turn her head against the neurologist's hand while the sternocleidomastoid muscle is palpated. The patient is also asked to shrug her shoulders while the trapezius is palpated.

The hypoglossal nerve (XII) is examined by asking the patient to stick out the tongue, to move the tongue in and out rapidly, and, finally, to wiggle it from side to side. Additionally, the patient is asked to roll the tongue upward and downward. Finally, the patient is asked to lick her lower lip.

These procedures are not a comprehensive assessment of all functions associated with the cranial nerves. Some of the functions, such as the vestibular functions associated with the acoustic nerve, require special equipment. Other functions, such as the sensory functions associated with the vagus, are too difficult to assess clinically. However, these procedures will provide the neurologist with an idea of the relative integrity of the cranial nerves. If the evaluation results in the identification of deficits or if functions are suspected of deficit, more rigorous evaluation may be performed.

Tests of Sensation

The sensory evaluation has been described as the most difficult and least reliable portion of the neurological assessment. This part of the evaluation starts by asking the patient about feelings of numbness, tingling, crawling sensations on the skin, coldness, or burning. The patient's sensitivity to tactile sensation is also evaluated. Light touches, hard touches, and pinpricks are used to determine whether the patient feels the stimulation. Patterns of sensory recognition versus absence of recognition are compared with the known distribution of sensory neurons in the dermatones. Sensitivity to vibration is also assessed. The patient's limbs will be moved passively, and the patient will be asked to state the direction of the movement. The blindfolded patient will be asked to identify the site of tactile sensation. Finally, two-point discrimination may be tested.

Tests of Strength and Tone

The motor system is assessed by examining muscle tone and strength. The neurologist will examine the muscle groups looking for fasciculation, atrophy, or tremors. The neurologist will also examine the patient for signs of abnormal tone, such as spasticity, rigidity, or flaccidity. The neurologist will also examine for signs of chorea, tics, tremor, or myoclonus, and will ask the patient to flex and extend her muscles both without resistance and when the neurologist provides resistance contrary to the movement. Here, the subjective nature of the exam is apparent, as the neurologist has to make a decision as to whether the motor strength exhibited by the subject is adequate or weak. Somewhat less subjective is the decision of whether strength is asymmetric.

Reflexes

Testing for certain reflexes is part of the evaluation of cranial nerves. However, some reflexes are not covered by the examination of cranial nerves, and need to be examined separately. The reflexes are divided into deep and superficial reflexes. The deep reflexes are tested by tapping a certain area of the body while that part of the body is relaxed. The speed and the strength of the reflex are compared with reflexes seen by the neurologist in other individuals. The deep reflexes include (with their normal responses) the biceps (contraction of the biceps), the brachioradialis (flexion of the elbow and pronation of the forearm), the triceps (extension of the elbow), the patellar (extension of the knee), and the Achilles (plantar flexion of the foot).

The superficial reflexes are tested by stroking the skin with a pointed object. The superficial reflexes include (with their normal responses) the upper abdomen (umbilicus moves up and toward the area being stroked), the lower abdomen (the umbilicus moves down), the cremasteric (the scrotum elevates), the plantar (the toes flex), and the gluteal (the skin tenses at the site of the stroke).

There are still other tests for pathological reflexes. These tests are for reflexes that were appropriate at an earlier age of development, but that should not be present in the healthy adult individual. These include the Babinski reflex, in which the lateral aspect of the sole is stroked. The abnormal response is an extension or dorsiflexion of the big toe and fanning of the other toes. In the Chaddock reflex, the lateral aspect of the foot below the lateral malleous is stroked. The abnormal response is an extension or dorsiflexion of the big toe with fanning of the other toes. The abnormal responses for the Oppenheim and Gordon reflexes are the same, although the stimulation changes. The stimulation for the Oppenheim reflex is stroking the anteromedial surface of the tibia. For the Gordon reflex, the stimulation is a firm squeeze of the calf muscles.

Following the completion of the neurological examination, the neurologist may order further tests and lab work to provide more information before establishing a firm diagnosis. However, the further work is usually needed only to determine a differential, the alternatives of which have been reached by use of the neurological examination.

NEURODIAGNOSTIC TECHNIQUES

If the neurologist suspects the presence of a neuropathological condition, she may order a more extensive workup of the client. Depending on the problem, several alternative procedures may be used. To acquaint the general clinician with some of these procedures, we will now give brief descriptions of the procedures and the circumstances under which they might be useful.

Electroencephalography

The electroencephalograph is a means of evaluating the electrical processes in the brain. There are several types of EEG available. The most common type involves the use of surface electrodes to record the electrical activity at several sites on the scalp. Another type involves nasopharyngeal leads to record the electrical activity. Nasopharyngeal leads are used to record electrical activity that has its origins in the basal aspect of the frontotemporal areas; however, they are rarely used because of the discomfort caused to the patient. EEGs can be taken when the patient is awake or asleep. Because sleep deprivation tends to accentuate EEG abnormalities, the EEG is sometimes recorded under those conditions. The EEG can be useful in the diagnosis of seizure disorders, but many patients with seizure disorders may have normal EEGs when they are not exhibiting seizure behavior. However, the presence of slow wave abnormality can be supportive of a diagnosis of a seizure disorder. In other words, the absence of abnormal wave form activity will not rule out a seizure disorder, but the presence of such activity can support the diagnosis of a seizure disorder. Other metabolic and systemic diseases can result in abnormal background activity. Large tumors or cerebrovascular lesions may result in focal signs in the EEG. The EEG can be useful in the diagnosis of encephalitis, degenerative processes, and metabolic encephalopathy. More recently, the quantitative EEG (QEEG) evaluates electrical activity on multiple sites in order to determine differences in brain activity (hypo- or hyperactivation).

Average Evoked Potentials

The average evoked potential (AEP) is a variation of the EEG. In the AEP, the patient is given some form of stimulation, usually auditory, visual, or somatosensory. The EEG in response to the stimulation is recorded over several sites and averaged into a single wave. The AEP allows the neurologist to measure the time it takes to process the stimulation, therefore facilitating estimates of conduction time. The AEP is useful in the diagnosis of demyelinating diseases, but the utility of AEPs for other disorders is not as well established.

Brain Electrical Activity Mapping

Brain electrical activity mapping (BEAM) is a technique that is used to assess differential levels of activation in the brain during a given task. In this technique, 20 electrode leads are attached to the surface of the scalp, similar to the procedures used for EEGs. However, with BEAM, the information from the leads is used to estimate the activity in adjacent brain areas that are not directly measured. This is accomplished using a regression procedure to predict activity in a nonmeasured area by using the values obtained at the three closest leads and the distance of the area from the leads. This information is computer analyzed, and the output is a three-color map of relative levels of activation in different areas of the brain. The BEAM procedure can be used in either a process EEG methodology or a discrete-event-evoked potential methodology. Although relatively new and somewhat experimental, BEAM has been reported to be useful in the identification of pure dyslexia (Duffy, 1981), dementia (Duffy, Albert, & McAnulty, 1984), and in epilepsy, cerebral infarctions, tumors, and learning disabilities (Duffy, 1982).

Clinical Magnetoencephalography

Another technique used to examine neuronal activity is clinical magnetoencephalography (MEG). MEG examines magnetic fields created by small electrical currents from the brain. Superconducting quantum interference devices (SQUIDs) are used to measure MEG. The distribution of the electrical currents is superimposed on MRI (described below), called magnetic source imaging (MSI). MEG and MSI can be used for the evaluation and treatment of epilepsy patients (Baumgartner, Pataraia, Lindinger, & Deeke, 2000; Moore, Funke, Constantino, Katzman, & Lewine, 2002; Pataraia, Baumgartner, Lindinger, & Deecke, 2002).

Skull Radiographs

Skull radiographs are often used to determine the presence of structural deficits in the head. Although in the past, skull radiographs have been used to diagnose degenerative disorders, tumors, inflammatory conditions, and even Cushing's disease (by documenting the thickening of vertebral endplates), they have been supplanted by the CT scan. However, skull radiographs are still useful in the evaluation of the acute effects of trauma.

CT Scan

The CT scan is actually a series of radiographs that are taken at different levels, or slices, of the brain. The results of each set of radiographs are fed into a computer that uses an algorithm to combine the different exposures into representations of the relative densities of structures in the brain. The CT is useful in the diagnosis of structural abnormalities such as tumors, cerebrovascular lesions, cerebral atrophy, and congenital anomalies. By first introducing a contrast material into the vascular system of the brain, the CT can be used to help differentiate between cerebral hemorrhage and edema. The use of contrast medium can also be helpful in determining the nature of a lesion (e.g., whether it is a glioblastoma or meningioma).

Regional Cerebral Blood Flow

Some neurological problems are metabolic rather than structural. In these cases, the neurologist may order a regional cerebral blood flow (rCBF). Although this procedure has shown promise in research settings, it has not been uniformly adopted in clinical settings. There are multiple methods, but the most common one is to have the client breathe oxygen that has been labeled with radioactive Xenon. To meet the metabolic requirements of brain activity, the oxygen travels to the areas in the brain that are being used. Multiple radioactivity monitors positioned on the client's scalp record the relative metabolic activity in these areas. In this way, areas of decreased metabolic activity can be identified.

Positron Emission Tomography Scans

Positron emission tomography (PET) scans are a method by which an indication of the functional activity of regions of the brain is obtained. The PET scan has largely superseded the rCBF in many research settings. The PET scan technology involves having the subject ingest a small amount of radioactively labeled glucose, and then engage in some cognitive activity. The brain areas with greater glucose use will show higher levels of the labeled glucose. Another use of the PET, although one with fewer clinical implications, is to label certain neurotransmitter ligands radioactively, thereby allowing identification of the sites in the brain in which the transmitter is taken up by receptor sites.

Single-Photon Emission Computerized Tomography

Single-photon emission computerized tomography (SPECT) is gaining in popularity because it is much less expensive to use, and the technology is readily available in many hospitals. Here, a chemical known as technetium-99m hexamethyl propylene amine oxime (HMPAO) is given intravenously to the subject. Uptake of the HMPAO is affected by rates of perfusion, allowing the clinician to evaluate differences in metabolic activity in regions of the brain. Both high and low levels of blood flow can then be documented; however, measurement is in only relative levels. Absolute levels of blood flow cannot be determined. Clinical applications are still developing. Belanger, Vanderploeg, Curtiss, and Warden (2007) suggest that SPECT has promise in identifying mild traumatic brain injury (TBI), and Djaldetti et al. (2009) report that SPECT can be used to index the severity of symptoms in Parkinson's disease, but clinical applications are still in the future.

Magnetic Resonance Imaging

The acronym MRI resulted from public concern over an earlier term for this procedure—namely, NMR, or nuclear magnetic resonance. Because that first name resulted in concern over "nuclear" activity in a hospital, the name was changed. MRI does not involve "nuclear" activity. It is based on the fact that nuclei spin, creating a magnetic field. Each type of nucleus has a particular spin with a signature magnetic field. When placed in a larger, stronger magnetic field, these nuclei will "hum" at an identifiable frequency. When a similar magnetic frequency is introduced, the nuclei absorb the energy and release this energy when the larger magnetic field is turned off. The strength of the signal sent out following turning off the larger magnetic field is proportional to the number of protons in a given area. By inducing various magnetic fields and turning them off, one can determine the relative amount of particular collections of protons. A computer can combine this information into "pictures" of the boundaries between different types of material that have different types of nuclei. The MRI procedures have been shown to be extremely useful in the diagnosis of multiple sclerosis, but other uses are experimental. Although, at first, it was hypothesized that the MRI would make the CT obsolete, at least one study has demonstrated the superiority of the CT in diagnosing acute subarachnoid or acute parenchymal hemorrhage (Snow, Zimmerman, Gandy, & Deck, 1986). In recent years, we have seen the advance of MRI applications and technology. For example, by comparing two serial MRI scans, one under resting conditions and one under conditions in which the subject is engaged in some cognitive activity, the examiner can de-termine relative blood flow and thereby provide a measure of functional activity in regions of the brain. Currently, the most frequent use of MRI is to determine structural anomalies or intracerebral bleeds.

Functional Magnetic Resonance Imaging

A more recent advancement is functional magnetic resonance imaging (fMRI) or functional MRI. Here, the MRI technology is used to measure activity across time and differences in regional brain activation. Because activation of brain cells involves the blood supply of glucose and oxygen, differential activation will result in systematically varying magnetic resonance values. When that data is analyzed using some form of time series analysis, patterns of activation may be uncovered. Clinical use is limited, and fMRI has greater application in research settings. The power of the technique can be seen in the wide applications to various research questions. Eisenberger, Lieberman, and Williams (2003) showed that the emotional experience of social rejection can be mapped with fMRI. Greene and Paxton (2009) showed that the neural activity associated with moral decisions can be indexed using fMRI. However, commercial and clinical use is increasing. Bernat (2009) discusses uses of the fMRI in diagnosing the persistent vegetative state versus deep coma. The fMRI results could potentially be used to identify reduced activation of different brain regions. Newsome et al. (2008) demonstrated that TBI may result in overactivation of certain frontal and prefrontal regions during performance of working memory tasks.

Newsome et al. (2009) showed that fMRI is sensitive to the increased activation brought on by administration of methylphenidate when individuals with TBI are engaged in tasks that require working memory.

Cerebral Angiography

Cerebral angiography is a radiological technique for visualizing the vascular system of the brain. In this technique, a small amount of radiopaque dye is introduced into the bloodstream via the artery that is in question. Following the injection of dye, a series of quick x-ray exposures are taken. Each successive exposure documents the progress of the dye through the artery. In this way, occlusions and other vascular abnormalities can be detected. Cerebral angiography can be useful in the evaluation of possible arteriovenous malformations, aneurysms, vascular tumors, and occlusions. It is generally used when other diagnostic techniques have not been successful, because of concerns about the amount of radiation to which the patient is exposed, because of the possible irritation from the contrast material, and because of the possibly painful nature of the procedure.

Lumbar Puncture

In some cases, the neurologist may want to examine the composition of the cerebrospinal fluid. In this procedure, the patient is placed on his side, and his lower back is prepped. The patient is instructed to arch his back as he draws his knees toward his chin. A local anesthetic is given and a needle is inserted, usually in the fifth lumbar interspace. The needle is pushed into the patient until it punctures the dura. The pressure is monitored, and then a sample of cerebrospinal fluid is drawn. The fluid can be tested for total protein, immunoglobulin, sugar content, the presence of bacilli, or the identification of malignant cells. This procedure has possible side effects of nausea, extreme headaches, dizziness, or neck pain. Therefore, it is used sparingly.

CONCLUSIONS

Although the neurologist and the neuropsychologist are both interested in CNS function, the evaluations used by the two types of professionals vary. The neurologist is less likely to use standardized behavioral tests such as those used by psychologists. The neurologist is more likely to be interested in cranial nerve function than is the psychologist. However, there are many points of overlap in the structure of the two types of evaluations.

Like the neuropsychological evaluation, the neurological evaluation is a series of assessment techniques that are usually conducted in a hierarchical fashion. The first components of the evaluation involve a complete history and a clinical evaluation of cranial nerves and gross corticobehavioral functioning. If the neurologist suspects dysfunction, but is unable to diagnose the exact condition, additional neurodiagnostic lab work may be ordered. The decision to pursue further evaluation is determined by the need for more information and the likelihood that the further tests will provide the necessary information.

4 The Neuropsychological History

A careful clinical interview examining the patient's history is the most powerful weapon in the arsenal of every clinician, whether generalist or specialist. Brain–behavior relations are extremely complex, and involve many different moderator variables, such as the age, level of functioning prior to current difficulty, and the amount of education. Without knowledge of values for these moderator variables, it is virtually impossible to interpret even specialized, sophisticated test results. The neuropsychological history is designed to obtain specific information regarding these moderator variables, as well as providing information related to risk factors, such as exposure to neurotoxins.

For example, although a *Wechsler Adult Intelligence Scale–IV* (Wechsler, 2008) full-scale (FS) IQ of 100 is considered average, obtaining a *WAIS-IV* FSIQ of 100 tells us nothing about the possibility of acquired brain impairment unless we know whether this represents a change in the level of functioning for the individual under consideration. If a clerical worker presents with a FSIQ of 100, we might conclude that there have been no changes in general intellectual functioning. However, if an engineer presents with an FSIQ of 100, we would want to investigate the possibility that the score represents a decline in general intellectual functioning.

Research studies frequently attempt to diagnose individuals simply on the basis of single test scores. This type of research can be useful in the evaluation of the diagnostic accuracy of tests, but these tests were not designed to be used in that fashion for clinical purposes. This sort of research, by its nature, attempts to isolate components of variables to examine them more carefully. Test scores are the most easily quantifiable components of test performance, and as such, are often used as variables in the evaluation of the validity of tests. From a practical standpoint, the classification of individuals as brain-impaired simply on the basis of test scores is a simplistic and dangerous practice. The data from tests should always be integrated with information obtained through a clinical interview, information regarding the appearance of the person, and information regarding the qualitative aspects of performance.

Specialized fields have developed specialized interview techniques and questions. The general interview and the specialized interview are similar. They differ in the relative emphases placed on types of information and in the types of questions asked. In the specialized neuropsychological interview, emphases are placed on investigating those variables that have been implicated in the relations between organic substrate and behavioral manifestations.

APPEARANCE OF THE SUBJECT

The generalist clinician is already trained to pay close attention to the physical appearance of the subject. The specialist is further equipped with a set of definitions for terms that are used to describe abnormal aspects of appearance. There are multiple reasons why a subject may present an abnormal appearance, but when used in conjunction with the history and the test results, information regarding the appearance of the subject can be an aid in diagnosis or in the decision to refer to a specialist. In each case discussed here, it is not recommended that the generalist try to interpret the observations. Instead, observations of abnormalities should be used in the decision to refer, and such information should be passed along in the report to the specialist to whom the referral is made.

The evaluation of the patient begins when he or she walks in the door. Is the patient alone or accompanied? If he or she is alone, does the patient possess enough memory skill to be able to remember the correct time and place of the appointment? Can the patient ambulate under his or her own power? Does the patient possess enough integrity of the visual–spatial system to find the location of the office accurately? Questioning the patient can help determine whether the subject was able to navigate public transportation or the use of a private automobile to arrive at the evaluation.

The dress and hygiene of the subject can help the clinician to determine the level of recent attention to grooming. There are multiple reasons why an individual may show signs of personal neglect in physical appearance; depression and apathy are two common causes. Personal hygiene is also a reflection of cultural background. Although not all patients will share the clinician's sense of fashion or of usual, everyday hygiene, most people will share the value of appropriate grooming before coming in for an appointment with a health care professional.

Although rare, a readily observable pathognomic sign of organic impairment can be seen in the individual who dresses carefully on one side of the body, but ignores the other side. This form of *unilateral neglect* will manifest itself in not properly buttoning or fastening clothes on one side of the body, or in men, in not shaving one side of the face. Somewhat more commonly, an individual may have poor hygiene over the whole body, but may not express awareness that something is amiss. This can be useful information, particularly if it can be ascertained that this is a recent development. Either of these observations may alert the clinician to the need for a more intensive mental status examination (MSE) and ultimate referral to a specialist.

LANGUAGE ABNORMALITIES

When the patient enters the office, observations can be made regarding his capacity to initiate an interaction. Does the patient spontaneously introduce herself? How are questions answered? Does the patient answer with single-syllable responses or is there amplification of the answer? If the patient answers with monosyllables, can he be encouraged to expand on his replies? Or does the patient become tangential when answering questions? What is the level of fluency? What is the apparent level of vocabulary? If there are questions regarding the vocabulary or fluency, a short standardized test such as the Vocabulary subtests of the *WAIS-IV* or the Peabody Picture Vocabulary Test–4 (Dunn & Dunn, 2007) can be given, supplemented by the Controlled Oral Word Association Test. *Dysfluency, dysartbria*, or other mispronunciation and abnormal word usage are important signs of a possible aphasic disorder. If there are long latencies in answering questions, special focus on the Attention and the Language portions of the MSE may be warranted. Informal observation of language can help with determining organic etiology of problems as well as general verbal abilities.

MOTOR ABNORMALITIES

Can the patient enter the room with the effortless ease that we associate with the absence of impairment? What is the general quality of physical movement? Is the gait normal? Does the patient move readily in a straight line, or does she walk at an angle? Can the patient walk around obstacles or does she bump into walls or into the furniture? Can the patient slow down and speed up her rate of movement in response to the requirements of navigation, or are changes in velocity jerky and abrupt? Are leg movements easy and free, or does walking appear to be an activity that requires much effort? Do the arms swing freely with the movements of the legs? Or is there either an excess arm movement or a tendency to keep the arms straight at the sides? Do the feet have a tendency to drop and point toward the ground when they are lifted in the walking movement, or are they kept relatively parallel to the ground, as is normally the case?

Observations of the quality of movement should continue throughout the evaluation. Because many of the procedures used in the MSE have motor components, many of these same questions should be asked when the patient is required to write or draw. Additionally, certain types of movement have implications for the diagnosis of neurological and neuropsychological disorders. *Tremor* may be noticed either when the patient is at rest or when the patient is asked to perform some motor activity. The conditions under which tremors occur should be carefully noted. *Intentional tremors are more likely to be due to lesions near the motor strip, whereas at-rest tremors are more likely to be due to subcortical lesions. In either case, referral to a neurologist may be indicated.*

The clinician should be alert for signs of a tic or other abnormal movements. Additionally, the clinician should note whether the tic occurs regardless of the situation, or whether the tic's occurrence or rate is affected by requests to perform some activity or when an emotionally charged topic is discussed. *Choreiform* movements are rapid, repetitive, stereotyped, purposeless movements that involve larger groups of muscles than do tics. The whole lower portion of a leg or an arm may be involved in a choreiform movement. The clinician must be observant, because a patient may have developed compensatory mechanisms to hide the choreiform activity. For example, one patient developed a habit of scratching behind his neck to hide the fact that he had a choreiform movement that involved rapidly lifting his right arm behind his head. *Athetoid* movements are another motor abnormality. In athetoid movements, there is an undulation of muscle groups. These may appear graceful, but they are involuntary and nonpurposeful, just as are the general choreiform movements.

There is also a class of movement abnormalities that have as their root the word "tonia." In general, these refer to disturbances in the tonic level of muscle activity. *Hypertonia* refers to a state of sustained high muscle tension. *Hypotonia* is a state of low muscle tension. The extreme instance of this condition is *atonia*, which literally means a lack of muscle tone. Patients with this condition would be unable to come to an office for an outpatient appointment, but they might be seen in inpatient settings. The patient may also show signs of *dystonia*, an involuntary motor activity that is slower and more sustained than choreiform activity. In addition, dystonia will usually contort the entire area of the body that contains the affected muscle group.

As well as abnormalities of tonic muscle condition, there may be signs of abnormalities of the level of muscle activity. For example, a patient may show signs of *akinesia*, which is a lowered level of muscle activity. Or there might be *akathisia*, which is motor restlessness, as shown by pacing or continual movement associated with subjective reports of restlessness. For each of these conditions, as well as for the conditions discussed previously, the reader is referred to chapter 1, which contains definitions of neurological and neuropsychological terms.

Abnormalities of symmetry can refer to either tonic muscle condition or to motor activity. However, these have different etiologies. For example, facial asymmetry may refer to asymmetry of the resting condition of the face, in which case, one side of the face may seem to droop, as in drooping eyelids (ptosis) or drooping at one corner of the mouth. Or there may be asymmetrical motor weakness, noticeable when the patient is asked to perform a movement such as raising his eyebrows or smiling. Additionally, the clinician should be alert as to whether the asymmetry occurs during voluntary movements (such as during response to a command) or with involuntary movements (such as those associated with spontaneous expression of emotions). One should also assess whether the upper part of the face, the lower part of the face, or both areas are involved. *When the right side of the face exhibits weakness, the clinician should be alert for the existence of other symptoms that are associated with left frontal lesions, such as right arm weakness and difficulty in producing fluent speech.*

ESSENTIALS OF OBTAINING THE HISTORY

In addition to the observation of the patient's behaviors, the clinical interview will also provide useful information. The overt purpose of the clinical history is to obtain information that can be used in determining a diagnosis and making recommendations, such as deciding whether to refer to a specialist. There are a series of questions that can be asked to obtain the necessary information. In effect, the patient tells us information with her verbal answers and with her associated behaviors. The earlier discussion in this chapter has focused on deriving information from the associated behaviors. We now concentrate on the types of verbal information that can be elicited from the patient.

It is critical to first establish a form of rapport with the patient. Patients are usually put off by the clinician who immediately starts asking questions. However, some balance needs to be struck, because the clinician wants to communicate the message that she recognizes the situation as a professional exchange. The clinician can greet the patient in a warm manner with a small amount of pleasant small talk, but only until the patient begins to feel at ease. It is helpful to begin the interview with straightforward, nonemotionally charged factual information to further allow the patient to adjust to the situation and to the clinician. For example, we suggest that the clinician briefly address the issue of confidentiality. Although there is no need to concern the patient unduly regarding the limits of confidentiality, it is preferable to describe the legal limits of confidentiality before the issue arises from the patient's verbalizations. This is especially true for those patients who are court-referred, or who may be involved in legal difficulties.

Identification of the Patient

The first few questions should relate to basic identifying information pertaining to the patient. The clinician can ask for the patient's name, phone number, date of birth, identified ethnicity, nationality, and country of origin. One can neither assume nationality nor country of origin. In northern cities in the United States, accents may vary little across the Canadian–U.S. border. In the Southwest, U.S. citizens who grew up in bilingual households may exhibit Hispanic accents. Knowledge of the nationality of the patient and the patient's parents can help in interpreting data regarding the use or pronunciation of verbal material. If the country of origin is different from that of the current nationality, the clinician should determine how long the patient has been in the country. The language that was used in the household of origin should also be determined. This should be done for all patients who report recent familial migrations to this country. All of these factors may affect a patient's performance on neuropsychological screening measures. Foreign origin or familial bilingualism reduces the diagnostic importance of poor performance on tests of language skills.

Current Complaints

After identifying who referred the patient for the evaluation, next, the clinician should inquire as to the history of the current disorder. It is important to pay attention to not only what the patient reports, but the way the information is presented. Does the patient recognize the problem, or did he or she come into the clinic because of complaints from others in the environment? It is important to gather the information from the identified patient prior to obtaining collateral information, if the patient is accompanied to the evaluation by a family member or friend. This helps not only to develop rapport, but to gain a better understanding of the patient's insight into the difficulty.

Obtaining information from the patient or family about his ability to perform daily activities of independent living is helpful in diagnosis. For example, examining the patient's ability to safely drive, consistently bathe, take medicine, tend to the finances, cook, and so on can help in clarifying the severity of functional disabilities. This information may assist in determining whether objective memory complaints meet criteria for mild cognitive impairment (MCI) rather than a dementia disorder.

It is important for the clinician to probe for related symptoms. A patient may withhold information not out of a desire to mislead, but because he or she is unaware of the importance of "trivial" symptoms (e.g., "trivial thirst"). For example, recent increases in thirst and in frequency of urination may indicate the onset of diabetes in patients who have initially come in with complaints of irritability, fatigue, or attention difficulties. In this instance, if the patient has not had a recent appointment with her primary care physician, a referral is necessary.

For all symptoms, the clinician should inquire as to when the symptoms first occurred, whether the quality and severity of the symptoms have changed over time, and the effect of these symptoms on the everyday functioning of the patient. Do others complain of the problem more often than the patient does? How was the problem first noticed?

The clinician should also try to ascertain the extent to which the current level of symptoms represents a change. If a change has occurred, the clinician should ask whether the changes have been slow and gradual, or abrupt. This can be important information in determining the differential diagnosis. *If the changes have been abrupt and no traumatic event such as a blow to the head can be documented, then the hypothesis of a cerebral vascular accident should be considered.* Referral for an MRI of the brain may be helpful. Similar to the information provided by abrupt changes, the quality of slow changes can provide information for the differential diagnosis.

Slow, gradual changes may reflect the presence of a dementia process such as Alzheimer's disease. Slow, stepwise changes that consist of a series of abrupt, but minor, changes across different functions may reflect the presence of multi-infarct dementia. In multi-infarct dementia, the subject is more likely to first show an abrupt change in the ability to perform mental calculations, and then a week later, there might appear impairment in short-term memory, and still later, impairment in a discrete area of language skills. A history of this type is more common in the patient experiencing a series of small strokes in diverse areas of the brain, as compared with Alzheimer's disease.

A history of a series of discrete impairments that are temporary in nature may be the result of transient ischemic attacks (TIAs). *A person experiencing TIAs is at high risk for future strokes, and should be referred to a neurologist immediately.* Prophylactic treatment in the form of diuretics will often reduce the danger from either multi-infarct dementia or TIAs. People suspected of having Alzheimer's disease should also be referred to a neuropsychologist, neuropsychiatrist, or neurologist for further evaluation, but the element of time urgency is not as important as in the cases of TIAs and multi-infarct dementia.

Obtaining a history of the present complaints also involves investigating the environmental and behavioral concomitants of the patient's complaints. The interaction of the biological and environmental is likely to contribute to the difficulties that that patient is experiencing. However, the relative importance of these two variables will change from disorder to disorder, and from case to case. The clinician should determine the antecedents and consequences of the occurrence of the complaint, because symptoms may arise from varied causes. For that reason, it is critical that the clinician inquire as to whether the patient is involved in litigation or had legal problems of any type, as this may influence the appearance of symptoms.

In one case with which we are familiar, a patient's complaints of memory impairment occurred 3 days after his notification that the compensation board had turned down his request for benefits based on a claim of black lung disease. The notification included the information that the board did not consider the patient's degree of claimed impairment severe enough to warrant compensation. Whether the patient was deliberately trying to mislead the clinician, or did not mention his memory problem previously because he did not think it relevant to his application for benefits, is immaterial. The fact remains that the memory complaints were linked to the environmental event of the notice from the disability board, and any evaluation would have been incomplete without this information.

In another case, it was determined that a patient's complaints of distractibility and short-term memory impairment were usually preceded by arguments with her teenage daughter, who was dating a person whom the parents did not like and who was allowing her school performance to decline. Subsequent evaluations indicated that the patient's problems were secondary to anxiety and stress.

Family History

Another area of information that should be investigated is the family history. The patient should be asked about family history for psychiatric disorders, because many psychiatric disorders, such as schizophrenia and major affective disorders, have genetic components. The presence of family members with these disorders will help clarify the diagnosis of the subject. In a like manner, there are genetic components to several neurologic disorders. The report of family members who were diagnosed with Alzheimer's disease, hypertension, Huntington's chorea, or other related disorders should sensitize the clinician to the possibility that these disorders might be present in the patient. The clinician should also inquire whether family members died early, or whether there were family members who were mentally retarded or learning disabled. Not all patients will be able to recall this information. Therefore, it is a good idea to suggest that the patient check out the information with other family members. In most families, there is an "historian," usually a parent or grandparent, who can remember details about which the patient may have no memory or no knowledge. One can suggest to the patient that such a person be contacted to obtain a more complete history. Some patients may be sensitive about family history, especially as it pertains to psychiatric disorders and suicide. The clinician should exercise tact and good judgment in questioning for this information.

Prenatal History

A history of prenatal events is a vital part of the history of the individual with suspected cerebral dysfunction. Unfortunately, it is routinely neglected by many clinicians, or the information is unknown by the patient. When the information is obtainable, it can shed light onto possible etiology for current behavior. Fetal exposure to a wide range of toxins or infectious diseases can have severe effects on cognitive functioning later in life. The clinician should inquire whether the mother worked while pregnant and where this work was performed. Was the mother exposed to solvents, insecticides, or dyes? What was the mother's use of drugs during pregnancy? This applies to both prescription and recreational drugs. The case of thalidomide is only one example, albeit an extreme one, of the consequences of some drugs. Fetal alcohol syndrome is another example of how maternal drug use can affect later cognitive functioning. Prenatal maternal exposure to infectious diseases, such as German measles, can also affect the cognitive development of patients.

Complications in pregnancy can affect the cognitive development of the patient. The patient may not be an accurate historian for questions of this sort, and should be encouraged to obtain the information from another source. Birth complications should also be addressed. Was the gestational age normal, premature, or late? Were there complications in the use of an anesthetic during birth? What was the weight at delivery? Was the use of forceps required?

Early History

Information about early development may have been transmitted to the patient in the form of family stories, but these should always be verified whenever possible. The clinician can ask for permission to talk with a family member to corroborate information obtained from the patient. The ages at which developmental milestones such as sitting up straight, walking, and talking were reached are important information. The clinician will also want to know about early posture and gait of the developing patient. Whether or not the patient experienced febrile convulsions should be determined. The presence of early developmental abnormalities may mean that there is a neurological substrate to the patient's current complaints. This is not to say that all patients with early developmental abnormalities or delays will have psychological disorders, only that the presence of developmental abnormalities tips the scale in the direction of deciding on a referral to a neuropsychologist or neurologist.

Personal development should be investigated. Did the patient experience school phobias? Was the patient able to form friendships as a child? What was the quality of these relationships? In general, the degree and type of social behavior is useful information in conducting this type of evaluation. It can help provide an estimate of whether the current complaints are recent or long-standing. For example, if a patient reports that he had many childhood friends and was involved in intramural sports and other extracurricular activities, but currently lives alone and rarely goes out to socialize, we would hypothesize a change in social functioning.

An accurate academic history is necessary to interpret information from testing and other sources. It is not sufficient to inquire as to the highest grade completed. There are multiple reasons why a patient may have terminated school early. Especially for older patients from a rural background, quitting school to help support the family by taking a job would not necessarily reflect limited intellectual capacity. Again, especially in rural states, compulsory education is a recent legal development. Patients may have grown up in an environment in which education was not valued, and may have quit school because their peer reference group was doing the same thing.

Conversely, in recent times, we have witnessed the unfortunate phenomenon of social passing in school. Despite an inability or unwillingness to do the work necessary, the contemporary urban patient may have been passed on to the next grade and may even have obtained a diploma. In all of the preceding cases, information about the grades earned by the patient and the type of classes taken should be obtained. This information can be verified, with the permission of the patient, by contacting the school involved or by contacting the person who was responsible for supervising the patient during that time.

Occupational History

An occupational history is an extremely important aspect of this sort of evaluation. The occupation can give two types of information: an estimate of intellectual functioning and an estimate of social-behavioral functioning. These must be considered rough estimates, as many people are underemployed, that is, they may be employed at a position that requires less than their maximum level of skills. However, the type of job held can be used as a lower-limit estimate of intellectual functioning. For example, an individual who holds a job as a college professor of romance languages would be assumed to have a high level of intelligence and language skills. Complaints by this sort of person about problems with word-finding difficulties and paraphasias represent serious impairment in ability.

Different jobs require different amounts of interaction with others. For example, a person with a job as a receptionist can be expected to possess a certain level of social skills. For such a patient to experience irritability and impatience with people denotes change in the social functioning of the person. Other jobs, such as that of computer programmer, require little interaction with others, and these patients would likely exhibit fewer social skills. Many computer programmers and other solitary workers may have more than adequate social skills, but this fact cannot be as readily assumed as it can in more people-oriented jobs.

Certain jobs may also expose workers to conditions that put them at risk for different disorders. The clinician should check to see whether the patient's job required working in a foreign country in which exposure to infectious diseases might have occurred. A history of encephalitis or meningitis may account for later cognitive complaints. Other domestic jobs may involve exposure to chemicals that can have cognitive and behavioral consequences. Workers who are employed in factories that manufacture insecticides, fungicides, batteries, glass products, or solvents may come in with complaints of irritability, insomnia, memory loss, impaired concentration, muscle weakness, or other problems. Patients who come in with any of these complaints, and who report that they work in environments in which putative neurotoxins are manufactured or used, should be referred to a neurologist or neuropsychologist for further evaluation.

During the past 20 years, research has elucidated the effects of many industrial chemicals on central nervous system (CNS) functioning. The most infamous of these is mercury. The history of observed neurotoxic effects of exposure to mercury in the workplace dates to the Victorian period of Charles Dickens and Lewis Carroll. At that time, mercury was used to fix the soft felt used in the manufacture of hats. Many of the workers in these plants developed psychological and behavioral problems, including emotional lability, irritability, and illogical behavior patterns. At this time, we know that there are different effects for exposure to organic mercury and inorganic mercury. Exposure to inorganic mercury may result in complaints of anxiety, an unreasonable phobia for social gatherings, and disruptions in emotional functioning. Exposure to organic mercury, such as methyl mercury, may result in complaints of restlessness and in observations of slowed mental operations. Large, single doses can be fatal, as in the incidence of fatalities seen in Japan in the early 1960s (Minamata disease) or in Iran in the 1970s, when many people who ate bread made from grain treated with a methyl mercury compound died. However, even small levels of exposure over several years can result in the development of symptoms leading to referral to a mental health professional.

Other substances such as lead, arsenic, carbon disulfide, carbon monoxide, solvents, and manganese (Feldman, Ricks, & Baker, 1980) can also cause psychological and neurological symptoms. The presentation of symptoms may be either immediate or delayed. For example, dependent upon the amount of exposure, carbon monoxide poisoning may lead to immediate complaints of headache, dizziness, and confusion. However, it has also been associated with generalized brain atrophy with specific decrease in the hippocampus (Gale & Hopkins, 2004). As a result, a patient with carbon monoxide poisoning may not demonstrate cognitive decline in language and memory until several weeks later. Similarly, our understanding of the effects of chronic solvent exposure has increased. Neurocognitive studies have consistently demonstrated that patients exposed to solvents have problems with memory, learning, psychomotor speed, and attention (Ellingsen, Lorentzen, & Langard, 1997; Morrow, Ryan, Hodgson, & Robin, 1990; Morrow, Stein, Bagovich, Condray, & Scott, 2001).

As our understanding expands, it is clear that exposure to many neurotoxins can cause cognitive and behavioral decline. The clinician who suspects exposure to neurotoxins as an etiological agent should inquire about gradual changes in appetite, sexual functioning, sleep patterns, memory, and emotional behavior. There are many possible symptoms, including anorexia, incoordination, ataxia, hypertension, and perceptual disorders (O'Donoghue, 1985), and many different causes for any of these symptoms. However, if these symptoms can be reasonably associated with exposure to neurotoxins, a referral to a specialist who can arrange for a complete medical workup is indicated.

Sexual History

The next area to be addressed in the history is that of sexual functioning. In our culture, sexual behavior is considered private, and many patients may demonstrate a reluctance to discuss such matters. Therefore, it is a good idea to inquire about sexual functioning late in the interview, after the clinician has had a chance to develop a rapport with the patient. Asking these sorts of questions early in the interview may unnecessarily frighten off a patient from making a full disclosure of relevant information. The clinician would be well advised to maintain an objective, professional demeanor during these questions to reassure the patient of the clinical nature of these inquiries. Some patients may need to be encouraged to provide this type of information. However, the clinician should never make light of the patient's reticence or probe too hard, as this is likely to alienate the patient.

These questions should assess past, as well as present, sexual behavior. For women, one should inquire about the age of menarche and whether there are any past or present irregularities in the menstrual cycle. Not all women are uniformly regular in their menstrual cycles. However, any changes in regularity should be noted. In addition, the clinician can ask about abortions and the conditions under which these might have occurred. For men, questions should include the age at which puberty was reached. These can involve the age at which the patient's voice started to crack, or the age of the first nocturnal emission or the first orgasm by masturbation.

For both sexes, the clinician should ask about the first sexual interactive behavior and other historical aspects of sexual behavior. Taking information about current sexual behavior would be insufficient, because it would not allow the clinician to determine whether a change had occurred. The question of homosexual behavior should be broached with sensitivity, because of the values placed on this behavior by our culture. The presence of a history of promiscuous behavior, whether heterosexual or homosexual, can alert the clinician to the possibility of sexually transmitted diseases, many of which have CNS effects if not treated. In recent years, the understanding of cognitive effects of acquired immunodeficiency syndrome (AIDS) have increased.

Changes in sexual behavior can have important implications for the current diagnosis. Decreases in sexual performance may be related to infectious diseases or exposure to neurotoxins. Decreases in sexual desire may be related to affective disorders. Impotence in men is commonly related to a psychological reason; however, it is wise to first rule out a physiological etiology.

Increases in sexual behavior may reflect either a neurological or a psychological etiology. Hypersexuality, reports of lowered need for sleep, incidences of spending sprees, and periods of extreme elation are often associated with manic-type bipolar affective disorder. Frontal lobe injuries, such as those sustained in closed-head injuries, may result in inappropriate sexual behavior associated with impulsivity. Changes in sexual behavior are also associated with subcortical tumors. The presence of changes in sexual behavior is not always associated with neurological disorders. However, information about sexual behavior is so important in establishing the correct diagnosis that the clinician who sidesteps the issue because of his own squeamishness is doing the patient a disservice.

Medical History

A medical history is a necessary step in the initial evaluation of a patient. This investigation should include long-term, as well as recent, history. Many childhood illnesses have CNS effects that are not present in adults. An example of this is German measles, which can lower intellectual functioning in children. The clinician should inquire about the occurrence of diseases such as meningitis, encephalitis, and epilepsy. The clinician should also inquire whether the patient suffers from migraines or other headaches. Headaches may signal the presence of a vascular disorder or a tumor, especially if seen in conjunction with cognitive or emotional changes. There are many possible etiologies for headaches, but a medical evaluation is needed to provide the diagnosis.

Any form of surgery, but especially neurosurgery, should be completely documented. Hip and knee surgeries have also been implicated in memory decline 3 months following surgery in elderly patients (Koch et al., 2007). The clinician needs to know whether a general anesthetic was used and whether there were any complications of the surgery, such as respiratory arrest or subsequent infections. In cases of respiratory arrest, there may be later problems with memory or attention, and those sections of the MSE should be emphasized. Any report of a closed-head injury should be amplified with information regarding whether hospitalization was required, whether there was a loss of consciousness, the duration of such a loss, and whether the subject exhibited posttraumatic amnesia. The duration of the posttraumatic amnesia should also be documented. Finally, the clinician needs to determine whether any behavioral patterns were changed following the injury, and the duration of these changes. Subjects with closed-head injury often exhibit increased irritability and temper, as well as decreased levels of patience.

It is evident that the patient will be a poor historian, particularly in the case of closed-head injury. A person can rarely observe her own posttraumatic amnesia or loss of consciousness. Changes in behavioral patterns may also not be evident to the patient. Once again, the clinician needs to contact someone in the patient's environment who was witness to the events or who is able to comment on changes observed in the patient. We cannot emphasize enough the importance of corroborating information with a secondary informant in this and in other matters, such as the determination of developmental milestones.

As part of medical history, a review of sensory organ functioning is recommended. Finding out whether the patient has recently been evaluated for his/her vision and hearing can rule out the possibility of sensory decline causing cognitive decline. Further, a decline in the sense of smell is thought to be predictive of dementia, and at the very least, appears to be linked to MCI (Wilson et al., 2007). Numbness or tingling in extremities may also be suggestive of numerous disorders, including multiple sclerosis.

A psychiatric history should be taken from all patients. For most general clinicians, this portion of the history will not differ from the history that is usually taken. The first questions involve whether the person has experienced any problems in the past, the nature of these problems, and whether the person sought professional help for these problems. The clinician would be wise to remember that depression is most often first seen and treated by a general practitioner or family doctor, and that many people refer their psychological problems to a member of the clergy for assistance. The type of treatment applied and whether the patient felt the treatment was successful is important information. Unsuccessful counseling treatments for complaints of depressed affect may indicate an organic basis to the complaints. There is a big difference between the disorder that was successfully treated by pastoral counseling and the disorder that required long-term hospitalization. If the patient has experienced problems in the past, the similarity of these problems to the current complaints should be elucidated.

A history of suicide attempts should always be investigated, and the presence of past or present suicidal ideation or suicide attempts should be documented. If there were past attempts, the lethality of these attempts should be determined, as well as the occurrence of hospitalization following the attempts. Not all suicidal reports need to be a cause of immediately hospitalizing the patient, but all reports of suicidal ideation should be carefully evaluated. Furthermore, suicide attempts accompanied by hypoxia put a person at risk for the development of memory, attention, or abstraction deficits that should be examined in the MSE.

The use and abuse of drugs also needs to be investigated. In our culture, the values placed on drug use may induce the patient to underreport her incidence of drug use, just as the laws of our society may incline the patient to deny drug use. Drugs, including alcohol, have powerful CNS effects. The clinician needs to impress on the patient the need for a completely accurate account of drug and alcohol use. Even at that, it is probably safe to assume that the levels of use reported by the patient are an underestimation. If the abuse has not been long term, some of the neuropsychological complaints, such as impaired short-term memory and decreased attention and concentration, may subside if abstinence is maintained for a period of 6 months. Unfortunately, most patients do not see a clinician until the effects of their substance abuse have become more widespread, and, in some cases, permanent.

Determination of premorbid personality and behavior patterns is another area that requires corroborating information from a source in the patient's environment. Some patients will be able to accurately describe changes that have occurred since the onset of the problem. However, it is more likely that patients will underestimate the degree of change, or will deny that any change has occurred. In its most extreme form, this is a symptom known as *anosagnosis*, literally the inability to know one's impairment. Family members are good sources for this type of information, because they have usually seen the patient in many different situations across many developmental stages. Consistent changes are more readily noticed by them than by acquaintances. As mentioned earlier, changes in temper, impulsivity, or patience can follow neurological insult to the brain. The other extreme is also possible; patients may become more apathetic and withdrawn following a closed-head injury.

Human social interaction is a complex set of operations that require subtle perceptual mechanisms and higher order judgmental processes. If a person experiences a neuropsychological impairment in any of the cortical-behavioral skills required, he or she may withdraw from situations that require social interaction because of the confusion and embarrassment that these situations cause.

Forensic information also needs to be gathered in the history. Again, this type of information is sensitive and should be corroborated. The clinician should inquire for both present and past legal difficulties. A long history of legal scrapes may indicate long-standing adjustment difficulties. A current increase in legal problems may indicate recent neuropsychological impairment. For example, impulsivity subsequent to frontal lobe injury may result in an increase in "spur-of-the-moment" ill-planned illegal activity.

A woman who was referred to one of our labs was brought in by her adult children because she had had 5 minor traffic accidents in a period of 6 months. Testing revealed that despite the fact that she was able to conceal most symptoms from her children, she was suffering from a degenerative dementia. As another example, a farmer who developed a temporal lobe tumor started exhibiting irrational behavior. He took out a large loan, ostensibly to update his farm equipment, and was unable to account for the money at the end of 4 months, ultimately defaulting on the loan.

Current Situation

Current litigation should be determined. The potential award of large sums of money can be a powerful contingency in shaping the motivation of a patient. In these cases, every effort should be made to obtain the cooperation of the patient in obtaining factual information and optimal test performance. Similarly, the threat of a jail sentence can influence the behavior of a patient, making this sort of information invaluable to the clinician. Few patients are neuropsychologically sophisticated enough to malinger in a consistent and neurologically coherent fashion across a variety of tests assessing cortical-behavior skills. However, the determination of malingering on neuropsychological tests is a decision best left to the specialist.

Finally, the current living situation of the patient should be evaluated. Recent changes in living situation, such as being asked to move out of a spouse's residence, can reflect behavioral difficulties. Conversely, changes in the living situation of organically impaired individuals can result in an exacerbation of symptoms. This is most clearly seen in the case of Alzheimer's disease patients, who become confused and irritable when even small changes in daily routine occur.

CONCLUSIONS

As discussed earlier in this chapter, the history can be a potent instrument in the evaluation of neuropsychological disorders. However, its power increases with the level of knowledge and skill of the clinician. This chapter can be used as an outline for taking a history, but the use of this outline does not guarantee success. With practice and experience, the clinician will become more adept at using the history as a means of conducting a complete evaluation. Informed observation of language can help with determining organic etiology of problems as well as general verbal abilities.

5 The Mental Status Examination

The mental status examination (MSE) can be a powerful tool in the repertoire of clinicians. The utility of the MSE can be seen in its adoption by several different disciplines. There are many different forms of the MSE that have been developed for use in areas such as neuropsychology, neurology, clinical psychology, psychiatry, and general medicine. Forms of the MSE sometimes also vary by particular institutions. The MSE that will be presented here is not unique. Nor is this MSE a test, per se. This format is meant to be a guide for the clinician in developing his own assessment procedures. In order to enhance the utility and accuracy of this MSE, the clinician should record the results of patients who are assessed with this set of procedures. In that way, the clinician can develop local norms and develop more objective means of interpreting the results.

The goal of an MSE is to obtain information that can be used in an initial formulation of the patient's problems. Different forms of the MSE reflect the types of information that the different disciplines use in clinical practice. For example, the MSE used by neurologists may include testing the reflexes and cranial nerves of the patient. We do not recommend that clinicians use procedures with which they may be unfamiliar. The procedures presented here are ones that can be used by most individuals who have graduate training in clinical psychology.

The amount of information derived from an MSE and the utility of that information in arriving at a diagnosis are partially determined by the skill level of the clinician conducting the MSE. Conducting the MSE smoothly and quickly is a behavioral skill that can only be achieved via practice. However, the level of interpretation depends on the amount of formal training and supervised clinical experience of the clinician. We intend this MSE to be used as an initial screen in the decision to refer to a specialist. No clinician can ethically exceed his expertise by attempting to interpret beyond his level of training and experience.

This MSE is not intended to replace a comprehensive neuropsychological or neurological evaluation. If signs of organic involvement are present, or if the results of the evaluation are questionable, the patient should be referred to a professional specialist (neuropsychologist or neurologist) for a more complete evaluation.

When seeing a patient for the first time, a complete history should be taken, especially if the patient is self-referred. For most patients, the MSE will take between 30 and 45 minutes. However, the length of the MSE will vary with the degree of the clinician's suspicion regarding the existence of organic impairment. Any areas that provide evidence for the presence of impairment should be followed up. This is not to say that areas that are not suspected can be safely ignored. Patients may come in with one complaint, and on evaluation, may manifest other, different impairments. Patients, like the rest of us humans, are not always the most objective judges of their conditions. Alternatively, patients may not feel comfortable relating all of the details of their problems. All areas, therefore, should be sampled, but in-depth evaluations may be required only in a portion of the areas sampled.

There are several classes of patients who can be considered a priori candidates for the extended MSE. These include patients with documented central nervous system (CNS) lesions. The lesions can result from tumors, trauma (closed-head injuries or penetrating wounds as the result of automobile accidents, sporting accidents, barroom brawls, etc.), or cardiovascular accidents (stroke). Another group of patients who should receive the MSE includes those with suspected CNS lesions. Although there may be no medical documentation of these patients' problems, they may complain of dizziness, seizure activity, headaches, or they may report a history of untreated head trauma. Some of these patients may report a history of metabolic medical disorders, such as meningitis or poorly controlled diabetes.

Patients with a report of sudden changes in emotional status, behavior, or in everyday aspects of cognitive functioning are also candidates for the MSE. For these patients, the information is more likely to originate from a source other than the patient, such as a family member. There are many different reasons why sudden changes in behavior or emotional condition may occur. Obviously, many of these reasons are environmental, and a functional analysis can provide good information in determining the etiology of the changes. However, sudden changes can also be the result of unreported traumatic events. The patient may not initially report a blow to the head, especially if the blow did not result in unconsciousness, but careful questioning by the clinician can uncover this fact. Fast-growing tumors can lead to precipitous changes in behavior. When a tumor is the cause, these changes in behavior may be accompanied by discrete, focal impairment. Recent sensory impairment is often associated with organic involvement and any reports of sensory impairment should be followed with an extended MSE. Positive findings on the MSE indicate the need for referral.

Complaints of psychiatric symptoms should also be investigated with an MSE. There is a large body of evidence to suggest that some psychiatric disorders are associated with neuropsychological impairment. In fact, an important question that is often faced by clinical neuropsychologists in psychiatric settings is the differential diagnosis of such individuals. Conversely, patients with neurological impairment will often present with psychiatric symptoms. There is not a strict dichotomy between neurological impairment and psychiatric impairment. Humans are complex phenomena whose various systems interact. It is, therefore, important not to think of a patient as having one type of disorder, but rather to view the patient as an individual with certain skills and deficits. Some individuals may have greater degrees of neurological impairment or of psychological and behavioral abnormality, but a pure case is rare.

ESSENTIALS OF THE EXTENDED MSE

Remembering the variability of individuals can help keep the clinician from thinking that all patients with disorder X will exhibit symptoms Y and Z. Such a clinician not only misses the richness of clinical detail in each case, but also runs the risk of overlooking ancillary or seemingly unrelated symptoms and complaints.

To help the clinician organize his thoughts, observations, and procedures, the MSE can be conducted in a hierarchical fashion. For all of their diversity, modern theories of brain function share the notion of the brain as the locus of a system of interrelating cognitive processes that are organized in some form of a hierarchy. Starting at the simplest levels and working up through more complex levels can help streamline the procedure of assessment by ruling out certain areas for which patients' component skills have already been seen to be impaired. As an example, if the patient is unable to add or subtract single digits in her head, the clinician does not need to assess the ability of the patient to perform serial subtractions.

Level of Consciousness

The first area of brain function to be evaluated is the level of consciousness. If the patient is able to appear for an outpatient appointment, a certain level of consciousness can be assumed. However, for the inpatient patient, there is likely to be more variability in levels of consciousness. Although it is unlikely that psychologists who work in an outpatient clinic setting will see injured patients in the acute stages of their injury, this occurrence is much more likely for clinicians working in a hospital setting. Here, the attending physician may call for a consultation to help determine the level of cognitive functioning to obtain a baseline, to chart recovery, or to document level of functioning to aid in placement planning. Therefore, we start by discussing some of the methods for assessing lower levels of cognitive functioning and move upward in the hierarchy. There have been several systems for evaluating and reporting the level of consciousness. We review some of them in the following text.

Strub and Black (1993) suggest that the level of consciousness be classified according to a four-part Guttman-type scale. Patients are assigned to one or another of these categories by noting the patient's response to some form of stimulation. There is a wide range of possible stimulation techniques, and a probably even wider range of patient responses. Therefore, it is important that the clinician document what form of stimulation was employed and what the response of the patient was. Relevant dimensions of patient response include eye openings and other eye movements, the presence of eye contact, the amount and quality of movement of any body parts, whether the patient engaged in speech and what the quality and content of that speech was, and a description of what the patient did following the assessment—whether he went back to sleep, asked for medication or food, and so forth.

In the first category, *Coma*, the patient is not arousable. The patient remains unconscious regardless of what the environmental stimulation may be. A patient in this category will not respond to verbal stimulation or even to painful stimulation. An example of the clinician's documentation of such a case would be, "Patient did not respond to my entering the room or calling out her name. No response to pinching the upper part of the shoulder. Patient appears to be in coma."

In the second category, *Semicoma* or *Stupor*, the patient is unconscious when the clinician enters the room and does not respond to verbal stimulation. The patient in this category will respond momentarily to persistent stimulation. Methods for eliciting a patient's response here can include shaking the patient's shoulder or pinching a fleshy part of the patient. An example of documentation would be, "Patient responded to persistent shaking of his shoulder by mumbling and rolling over; did not regain consciousness."

In the third category, *Lethargy*, the patient will respond to stimulation, but only briefly before falling back into unconsciousness or sleep. An example of documentation would be, "Patient responded to my calling out her name by briefly opening her eyes. She was able to answer one question before falling back to unconsciousness. Could be reawakened by calling her name again, but repeated the pattern of losing consciousness after a short period."

In the fourth category, *Alert*, the patient can respond to environmental stimulation. She is able to answer questions and to interact with others. For psychiatric patients, interaction with others will be moderated by level of motivation. Paranoid patients may have the capability to interact with others but may choose not to do so. The clinician's judgment is important in such cases.

There are multiple reasons why the patient may behave in a particular manner following stimulation by the clinician. For example, lethargy may be secondary to a recent dose of pain medication. The clinician should, therefore, note the time of day when assessment was conducted, as well as the recent previous events. In inpatient settings, the nursing staff can be helpful in obtaining the relevant information.

The Glasgow Coma Scale

Another system of describing the level of consciousness is known as the Glasgow Coma Scale (Teasdale & Jennett, 1974), which we have already briefly discussed in chapter 1. The Glasgow Coma Scale was also developed as a Guttman-type scale. Patient responses are evaluated in three major areas, and the highest level of response for each area determines the Glasgow Coma score.

The first area of patient responses is that of motor responses. The highest level of response here is an ability to obey commands. The commands may vary along a continuum of difficulty and complexity, but should not be so simple as to be confused with a reflexive motor response. For example, when placing one's finger in the patient's hand, the patient may grasp the finger regardless of whether a verbal command to do so is given. Commands that are less likely to be confounded with reflexes include raising the arm, turning the head, or moving a major limb. Keeping in mind that such movements may also occur spontaneously, successfully completed commands should be repeated to assess the reliability of the results.

If the patient does not respond to verbal commands, one can apply a painful stimulus. One should be sensitive to whether any subsequent movement appears to be an attempt to move the limb from the painful stimulus or simply reflexive movement. The next lower level of motor response is the flexor response. In this response, the patient reacts to the clinician straightening her abducted limb by resuming abduction. The next lower level is extensor posturing, and the lowest level is no response.

Verbal responses constitute the second area of assessment in the Glasgow Coma Scale. At the top end of this scale, the patient is able to state accurately his name, the place where he is and why he is there, the city, year, month, date, and approximate time. Any inaccuracies in the patient's orientation should be noted.

The next-lowest level of verbal responses is known as confused conversation. In this condition, the patient is able to respond verbally to questions and to keep her attention on the clinician, but the verbalizations of the patient indicate that she is confused about the situation or about the question of the examiner. For example, one of our head-trauma patients was asked the question, "What is your son's name?" to which he replied, "1913." The patient was sitting up in bed, watching television, and appeared to be normal. Further questioning indicated that the patient thought that the soap opera on the television was some sort of game show for which he could not figure out the rules.

In the next-lowest level of verbal responses, inappropriate speech, the patient uses speech that is recognizable as words but that seems unrelated to environmental events. This speech appears to be random and is often loudly exclamatory or vulgar. In this level, the patient is unable to conduct a conversation.

The next-to-lowest level of verbal response is that of incomprehensible speech. In this category, the patient will exhibit groaning or other sounds that do not have semantic referents. In the lowest level, there is no sound produced via the speech apparatus.

The third area of responses relates to eye opening. Spontaneous eye opening consistent with the patient's sleep/wake cycle is the highest level of response in this area. There are no assumptions made regarding the level of attention here, or whether the patient is able to understand what is going on around her.

The next level of response in this category is eye opening in response to speech. Because of the difficulty in determining whether the patient is responding to a command to open the eyes or is merely responding to the verbal stimulation, the difference between the two is not scored here. The determination is made by whether or not the patient opens the eyes when speech, loud or otherwise, is produced by the clinician.

The next-to-last level is eye opening in response to pain. Here, the painful stimulus is best applied at a site distant to the eye. Reflexive responses in the ocular muscles to the pain may otherwise obscure the nature of the response. The last level is, of course, no eye opening.

Rancho Los Amigos

Still another scale that has been used to describe levels of arousal is the Rancho Los Amigos Scale. Actually, the Rancho Los Amigos Scale attempts to describe levels of cognitive functioning. Rather than assessing the level of functioning separately in different areas as the

Glasgow Coma Scale does, the Rancho Los Amigos Scale uses a unidimensional scale of generally increasing levels measured in different areas simultaneously. There are eight levels to this scale.

The first level is "No Response." Here, the patient appears to be completely unresponsive to any stimulation. The second level is "Generalized Response." Here, the patient may inconsistently react to stimuli. The reactions involve orientation responses and attempts to withdraw from a painful stimulus, but there is an absence of meaningful responses.

The third level is "Localized Response." Here, the patient may react in a meaningful way to a stimulus, but the response is delayed and may be inconsistent. Simple commands may be followed, but, again, this occurs in an inconsistent manner. In the fourth level, "Confused–Agitated," the patient may exhibit a fairly high level of activity, but she does not appear to be able to process information meaningfully. Often, aggressive behavior is present. The patient does not discriminate between persons and objects. Verbalization occurs for the first time here, but it is incoherent or inappropriate. In this level, the patient is unable to care for herself, although motor activity such as rocking or pacing may be present.

The fifth level is "Confused, Inappropriate, Nonagitated." Here, the patient is alert and can respond to simple commands consistently. However, she is unable to perform to complex commands. This patient is highly distractible and needs frequent redirection to remain on task. Memory is impaired, but the patient can usually recognize family members.

In the sixth level, "Confused–Appropriate," the patient demonstrates instrumental, means–ends behavior, but requires external direction for successful completion of most complex tasks. He can follow simple commands. This patient is oriented to time and place. Memory is still somewhat impaired. He is able to perform most activities of daily life with minimal supervision.

The seventh level is "Automatic–Appropriate." Here, the patient is able to perform most required activities, but goes through the behaviors in a seemingly automatic fashion. This patient has superficial awareness of her condition and exhibits poor judgment. Some of these patients may be appropriate for vocational rehabilitation.

In the eighth and final level, "Purposeful and Appropriate," the patient is alert and oriented. He is able to learn new skills and is aware of his current condition. He is able to perform most activities independently.

From examining the preceding levels, it becomes clear that not all patients will fit neatly into one of the levels. Individuals may be in one level for a given area of functioning and in another level for a different area. However, as a gross indication of the level of functioning, as well as of the extent to which independent functioning is possible, the Rancho Los Amigos Scale may be helpful.

ORIENTATION

Orientation is a term used to describe the accuracy of a patient's perception and understanding of the events surrounding him. Orientation is not a unitary construct, but is instead composed of different types. Commonly, these are referred to as orientation to person, place, date, and time. For most patients, these can be placed along a continuum of difficulty and seriousness, with lack of orientation to person being the most serious and lack of orientation to time being the least serious. In most situations, orientation is assessed by simply asking the patient her name, the place, the date, and the time. Orientation to the date can be further broken down into accuracy for year, season, month, day, and date. Despite its history as a usually informal assessment technique, there are a few standardized procedures available to assess orientation.

The Galveston Orientation and Amnesia Test (GOAT) was created to evaluate orientation in head-trauma patients and to chart changes as the recovery process progressed (Levin, O'Donnell, & Grossman, 1979). The GOAT is very short and consists of only 10 basic questions that cover orientation to person, place, time, and date, as well as questions regarding memory for events directly preceding and following the injury. It is scored not only for whether the answers provided by the patient are correct, but also for the degree of accuracy of the answer. For example, five error points are assigned if the subject is unable to recall what happened right before the injury occurred, and another five error points are assigned if the patient is unable to recall any events before the injury. The GOAT has been found to be related to Glasgow Coma Scale scores, to computed tomography (CT) results, and to eventual recovery outcome of the patient. Normative data, based on a sample of 50 patients, is also available (Levin, O'Donnell, & Grossman, 1979).

Benton, Van Allen, and Fogel (1964) have standardized an instrument that can be used to assess temporal orientation in both inpatients and outpatients. In this evaluation, the patient is asked to state the current date, the day of the week, and the time of day. Scoring is performed by assigning each patient 100 points and subtracting points for each error made. One point is subtracted for the day of the week for which patients are inaccurate (to a maximum of 3 points), 1 point is subtracted for each day of the month the patient is off (to a maximum of 15 points), and 5 points are subtracted for each month the patient is off (to a maximum of 30 points), with the exception that if the date is correct within 15 days, points are taken off for the date, but not the month. For example, if the correct date is March 7 and the patient replies, "February 27," points are subtracted for the incorrect date but not for the incorrect month. Ten points are subtracted for each year removed from the current year (to a maximum of 60 points), with the exception that if the patient response is within 15 days of the correct answer and the assessment occurs near the beginning or end of the year, no points are subtracted for the incorrect year. For example, if the date is January 12, 1988, and the subject replies "December 30, 1987," no points are subtracted for the year, although points are subtracted for the incorrect day. Finally, 1 point is subtracted for each ½ hour for which the patient is incorrect (to a maximum of 5 points).

The differential weights assigned to types of errors indicate that this Test of Temporal Orientation is sensitive both to the presence of error, as well as to the seriousness of the error. The performance of 110 medical inpatients without suspicion of organic mental impairment indicated that only 9% of the patients scored between 98 and 95 points, the remainder scoring higher. For the 60 cognitively impaired patients, 27% scored between 98 and 95 points, and 13% scored even lower. However, it must be pointed out that 458 of the cognitively impaired patients gave perfect scores on this assessment. Levin and Benton (1975) subsequently found that the Test of Temporal Orientation identified temporally disoriented patients about 1⅓ times as frequently as the standard neurological examination. Later, Natelson, Haupt, Fleisher, and Grey (1979) reported that normal patients with lower amounts of education tended to make more errors than did normal patients with more education. In this sample, 5% of the normal medical patients achieved scores lower than 97. Unfortunately, the authors do not report the actual score distribution, so it is difficult to tell what the scores of those lower subjects were. However, it appears safe to say that scores lower than 95 should be an indication that a more thorough evaluation is in order. It is important to remember that because 45% of the impaired subjects in the original sample gave perfect scores, this screening test should not be used to rule out impairment, but rather to indicate which patients are most appropriate for referral to a specialist. In general, significant disruption of orientation (i.e., year, month, and place) in the absence of a serious psychiatric disorder should be followed up with a more extensive MSE, as an eventual referral to a specialist.

ATTENTION

Once the level of consciousness has been assessed, the level of attention can be evaluated. Naturally, if the patient is unconscious, the assessment can terminate there. However, in the outpatient setting, attention is the first area likely to be assessed, especially if the patient is self-referred and the clinician is naive as to the condition of the patient. *Attention* is sometimes defined as the ability to attend to specific stimuli without distraction. The fact that the root (attend) is used in the definition speaks to the difficulty of defining such a term. Attending involves focusing one's perceptual mechanisms on a particular stimulus and actively processing the information. These are all private events. We can only assess attention by behavioral observation of the covert by-products of attention, by history, or by the use of procedures that require attention for their successful completion. An example of such procedures is the Digit Span portion of the *Wechsler Adult Intelligence Scale–Third Edition* (WAIS-III; Wechsler, 1997). (Other examples will be given later in this section.)

Vigilance is another term that is often invoked in a discussion of attention. Vigilance is usually used to describe a sustained period of attention, such as attention for 30 seconds. Vigilance figures heavily in the experimental literature. There are many procedures for assessing vigilance in the laboratory. There are discrimination paradigms, reaction time paradigms, and others that are not easily duplicated in a clinical setting. However, there are several procedures that can be used to assess vigilance in the clinical setting.

One of these procedures is the "Random Letters Procedure." To use this procedure, one must first have prepared a list of 75 letters in random order. One letter, say the letter C, should be repeated 10 times in the list. The clinician states the letters at the rate of three every 2 seconds, and instructs the subject to tap a pencil each time she hears the letter C. Subjects with unimpaired vigilance should be able to make no more than one error in a 30-second period.

One method of assessing vigilance or sustained attention for shorter periods is to have the subject listen to a series of taps that the examiner makes under the table or that the examiner has prerecorded. It is important that the subject not receive extra cues from visual information. The series of taps should vary in length from 3 to 15. Have the subject count the taps and report the number. A normal subject should not have more than minimal trouble with this task.

Attention can be assessed throughout the MSE by observing the ability of the patient to follow the course of the examiner's verbalizations. For example, if the patient often has to request that the examiner repeat questions, it may be an indication that the patient is having difficulty maintaining sustained attention. If the patient replies to questions with inappropriate answers, the examiner should repeat the question to make sure that receptive language impairment is not the responsible issue. For example, if in reply to the question, "How long have you lived at your current address?" the subject replies, "297 Spruce Street," the examiner can repeat the question. If the subject now replies, "About 2 years," the initial incorrect answer may reflect poor attention rather than a deficit in understanding verbal communication.

One aspect of attention relates to the ability of the subject to finish a mental operation that requires some thought. A procedure that can be used to assess this aspect is the use of serial subtractions. Tell the patient to start at 100 and subtract 7, then to subtract 7 from that number, and so on. Serial subtraction is a complex activity that requires arithmetic ability and memory as well as mental control, so impaired performance may not be specifically related to impaired attention. However, if impairments in the other skill areas can be ruled out, impaired attention may be the cause of impaired performance. Assessing the qualitative components of performance can also help in interpreting results from this type of assessment. People with lower education levels may perform correctly, but slowly. People with impaired arithmetic skills may perform at a reasonable rate, but their performance will be inaccurate. People with impaired attention will give a more variable performance. They will be slow and inaccurate. They may drift off, forgetting the task at hand. Or they may start the procedure, only to stop and ask the examiner what the question was.

Attention is also sometimes applied to the question of whether or not the subject is capable of attending to the entire perceptual field simultaneously. There are two general classes of disorders that impair this type of attention. The first, visual field cuts (sometimes called *homonomous hemianopsia* if the same side of the visual field is missing in each eye) are usually the result of a cerebral vascular accident. Unilateral neglect involves inattention to an entire side of one's perceptual field. These patients may read only the right side of a card with printed letters. In an extreme form of hemi-inattention, a patient familiar to us would dress only the right side of his body and would shave only the right side of his face. More often than not, a patient with this type of disorder will have a subtler presentation. Because of the strong contingencies usually present in the natural environment, people with this type of disorder will quickly develop compensating strategies, such as alternate visual scanning procedures. Assessment of these suspected deficits can, therefore, be tested using double simultaneous stimulation.

In double simultaneous stimulation procedures, first unilateral sensory stimulation is confirmed. This is accomplished by presenting stimulation (e.g., visual, auditory, or tactile) to only one side of the body. After single sensory reception has been verified, both sides of the body are stimulated at the same time.

To test the visual fields, one stands about 3 feet in front of the patient and instructs the patient to fixate on the examiner's nose. The examiner, then spreading his arms and pointing his fingers inward, will wiggle one or the other, asking the subject which finger is being wiggled. The arms are moved in a general circle around the subject's face. If the subject is unable to state which finger is being wiggled correctly, the examiner moves the finger in, reducing the size of the visual field until the finger movement is recognized. The examiner should try to ascertain that the subject remains fixated on the examiner's nose during this procedure, as lateral eye movements will invalidate the results. Finally, the examiner can alternate both fingers wiggling with only one finger moving to see whether the subject can identify movement on both sides of the body at the same time. Failure on this task is referred to as *suppression* by the neuropsychologist and *extinction* by the neurologist. Suppressions can occur across different sensory modalities.

Auditory unilateral inattention is tested by standing behind the subject (out of the subject's line of sight), and lightly but audibly rubbing one's fingers close to the subject's ears. First one side is tested and then the other, and then both simultaneously. Again, the subject is asked to identify the correct side of the body being stimulated.

Tactile hemi-inattention can be tested by lightly touching the cheek of a blindfolded subject with a cotton swab or the edge of a tissue, first one side and then the other, and, finally, both. Before using this procedure, it is important to first describe what will be done (i.e., "I am now going to touch you with the tip of a cotton swab"). This will help alleviate any anxiety caused by the blindfolding.

Unilateral attention deficits are almost always the result of localized lesions in the cerebral cortex. Patients who demonstrate this type of deficit should be referred for a complete evaluation. Generalized inattention has a wider range of etiologies. Inattention may be caused by lesions in either the ascending or the descending reticular activation system. Alternatively, it may be the result of bilateral frontal lobe lesions. Either one of these will usually be accompanied by signs associated with the particular etiology, and diagnosis of one or the other should not be done on the basis simply of inattention. Inattention may also be the result of diffuse metabolic disorders. Uncontrolled diabetes, thyroid conditions, liver dysfunctions, and vascular disorders are only a few of the possible metabolic causes of inattention. Finally, disturbances in attention can also be the result of a psychiatric disorder such as depression or schizophrenia. The generalist clinician should not try to diagnose the problem, but should instead carefully document the observations made during the evaluation so as to be able to pass the information along to the specialist.

LANGUAGE

Language functions are required for the patient to understand and respond to questions by the examiner in all sections of the MSE. Therefore, the assessment of language functions is not confined to a separate section of the MSE, although there are particular procedures that can be used to assess language functions in this part of the evaluation. At a most general level, language functions can be dichotomized into receptive language function and expressive language functions. Receptive language skills include the ability to perceive and understand language, whether it is communicated in an auditory/spoken modality or a written/visual modality. Expressive language skills also involve both auditory and written modalities. Both can be further broken down into symbolic and sensory/motor aspects. In keeping with the proposed hierarchical structure of the MSE, the assessment of language functions starts at a simple level and progresses to a more complex level.

First, to assess comprehension, give the subject a series of simple commands progressing to more complex commands. This sequence may be useful.

1. Please close both of your eyes.
2. Now open both eyes.
3. Raise an arm.
4. Raise your left arm.
5. Put your right hand on your left knee.
6. If today is Tuesday, raise both of your arms; otherwise, raise only your right arm.

The earlier in this sequence that the patient fails, the more likely there is a need for a referral.

Assessing the level of expressive language functions includes testing the ability to name an object from a picture. It must be remembered that this sort of task (confrontation naming) is also affected by the general integrity of the visual system. Peripheral visual impairment, as well as visual agnosia, must be ruled out before an interpretation of expressive speech impairment is reached. The clinician can obtain pictures of everyday objects that can be readily recognized. Mount these singly on index cards. Present them one at a time to the patient and ask her to name the object pictured. Note whether the patient is able to correctly name the item, or must instead describe its use. If the patient can name the object, note whether the pronunciation is correct. Keep in mind the regional differences in pronunciation that the patient might exhibit as a result of the location where the patient was raised. If the patient can neither name the object nor describe its use, she may have a visual agnosia, that is, an inability to recognize the meaning of visual information.

To assess the patient's basic levels of receptive and expressive language, one can start with a repetition task. Ask the patient to repeat what he hears. Give a list of words that progress from short, simple words to more difficult words. For example, state, "Repeat after me—one, top, pipe, basket, cabinet, affection, stentorial, pleurisy, Methodist." Next, give the subject a card on which the same words have been printed and ask the subject to read them out loud. A differential between performance on the repetition task and the reading task can help determine the type of deficit involved. Any mispronunciations or stumbling should be noted.

If the patient is able to repeat and read simple words, move to phrases, and finally, sentences. The following phrases can be given orally first and then on a printed card.

1. In good time.
2. Follow the leader.
3. A ferocious lion.
4. Coming at an inconvenient time.
5. The boy kicked the ball.
6. The pitcher wound up and threw the ball.
7. If ever the sky should turn green, you should seek shelter.

Here the examiner should pay attention to elements of speech regulation, as well as pronunciation. The ability to modulate speech tone may be impaired in some patients. These patients may demonstrate a monotone delivery, or, less commonly, may demonstrate abrupt and inappropriate changes in tone of voice.

To get an idea of the functional level of language skills, one can ask the patient to describe a picture that portrays more than one activity. Pictures of this sort can be found in popular news magazines and can be mounted on an index card. One can also ask the patient to describe his home (or job, hobby, or favorite television program). Here, the clinician is attentive to multiple aspects of language production. If the patient has gotten this far in the evaluation of language, the more important aspects involve the ability to string together words in a manner that makes sense, appropriately matching the tone of voice to the content of the speech and speaking in a smooth manner. Additionally, the clinician should note the latency between giving the command and when the patient starts to reply, as well as the relative richness or paucity of speech production. If there is low production, appropriate follow-up evaluation includes the use of the Controlled Oral Word Association Test or a vocabulary test.

The ability of the subject to write can also be assessed. Moving from simple words to simple phrases, the clinician can have the patient write from dictation and then copy from a printed card. The responses can be examined on the basis of spelling and legibility. Spelling errors should be evaluated in light of the patient's highest level of academic achievement. Legibility can be affected by motor problems that will be noticed in other parts of the MSE, as well as here.

MEMORY

Memory impairment is a common complaint, both for patients with primarily psychological problems, such as depression and anxiety, and for patients with primarily neurological problems. Memory disruption is such a common complaint, it was at one time thought that all acquired brain impairment would include disturbances in memory. Many early screening tests for organic impairment were tests of memory. An example of this is the Wechsler Memory Scale (WMS; Wechsler, 1945). David Wechsler originally envisioned the WMS as a test for general organic impairment. Influenced by equipotentiality theory, he hypothesized that all head injuries would result in some memory impairment. There are other memory screening tests available, and those will be discussed in the section on screening instruments.

Memory is a multidimensional construct, and patients may be differentially impaired for different types of memory. Different researchers have proposed different subdivisions of memory. Among the most common are (a) verbal memory—memory for words, phrases, and short stories; (b) visual memory—memory for designs and colors; and (c) spatial memory—memory for the position of objects. Additionally, there may be memory for musical tones, tactile sensation, and proprioceptive information.

It is possible to obtain an informal assessment of memory within the confines of the MSE. Clinical evaluations of memory have tended to divide the assessment of memory into three categories: immediate memory, short-term memory, and long-term memory. These terms do not carry the same meanings in the clinical setting as they do in the laboratory investigations of memory, and should not be confused with their laboratory and information-processing meanings. In the clinical setting, *immediate memory* refers to events and occurrences in the MSE itself. *Short-term memory* refers to recent daily events. *Long-term memory* refers to remote events.

Short-term memory is usually assessed with a repetition task. In keeping with the preceding discussion regarding different types of memory, the clinician may want to assess the different types of memory separately. A prepared list of four unrelated words is useful in this evaluation. The examiner can give the list "violin, door, grape, pencil" and then ask the subject to repeat the list. This same list can be used to evaluate the effect of delay with distraction on memory. The clinician could then continue the evaluation. After 5 minutes have passed, the patient is again asked for the list of four words. Any four unrelated words can be used; however, it is a good idea to write down the list first to guard against the clinician forgetting the list or confusing it with a list used with another patient.

Some patients who are impaired for unrelated words may have normal memory when the verbal material is contained in a meaningful context, such as a short story. To assess this, the clinician can type a short story (similar to that used in the WMS) on an index card. Read the story to the patient and count the number of concepts in the story that the patient remembers. This assessment can again be conducted after 5 minutes to assess the effects of distraction and delay.

Still another type of memory involves the association of items. A card typed with a list of five related and unrelated pairs of words can be used in this evaluation. This procedure is similar to the Paired Associates section of the WMS and the Paired Words section of the Randt Memory Test. If the clinician is sure that neither of those two tests will be used in a later evaluation of the patient, those lists may be used here. However, it is more prudent to compose one's own unique list, so as not to bias and possibly invalidate later evaluations. A possible list is "opera–singer, railing–paper, dish–supper, cabinet–tiger, bell–ceiling." Both words are given at first, with pairs separated by a 1-second delay. Then only the first word is given, and the patient is asked to provide the second word. By repeating this procedure until the patient is able to state each pair correctly to a maximum of five trials, one can also assess the learning curve of the patient. Most normal subjects should be able to achieve a perfect score within three trials. The fact that some of the words are related and some are not will allow the clinician to assess informally differential memory for meaningful and nonmeaningful pairs. It should be remembered that this is an informal assessment without a normative base and no statements regarding a diagnosis of memory impairment can be made without following the MSE with a standardized assessment.

Visual memory can be evaluated by showing the patient three pictures that can be clipped from a magazine and mounted on cardboard. The patient is then shown a series of six pictures, only three of which were included in the first series, and asked to identify which of the pictures he has seen before during the evaluation. Visual memory can also be assessed by showing the patient an abstract design such as the illustration depicted in Figure 5.1. Allow the subject to view the design for 5 seconds. Then remove the design and ask the patient to draw the design. Impaired performance can be the result of problems in visual–motor coordination as well as in visual memory, so a report of the results should stick to a simple description of the behavioral task that the patient was unable to do.

Visual–spatial memory can also be assessed using a hidden objects procedure. In the presence of the subject, hide four objects. After a delay of 5 minutes, ask the patient to point out where the objects are hidden.

Recent memory is usually assessed by asking the patient about some events in his day, such as what he had for lunch, or what color the waiting room furniture was. The clinician should not ask questions for which she does not know the answer. Doing so would negate the purpose of the question. Long-term memory is usually assessed by asking the patient autobiographical questions, such as asking him to state his home address during childhood, or what the name was of his fifth-grade teacher. Again, the clinician should know the correct answer for any questions asked. This can be accomplished by previously questioning a family member.

Impairment of immediate memory may be the result of lesions in the Sylvian fissure, or the result of a metabolic disorder, or the result of acute alcohol or drug intoxication. Disturbances of recent memory may be the result of subcortical lesions, especially lesions of the hippocampal region. Impairment of remote memory may be the result of frontal lesions or diffuse cortical dysfunction. Transient global amnesia may result from transient ischemic attacks and should be immediately followed up with a complete medical/neurological workup.

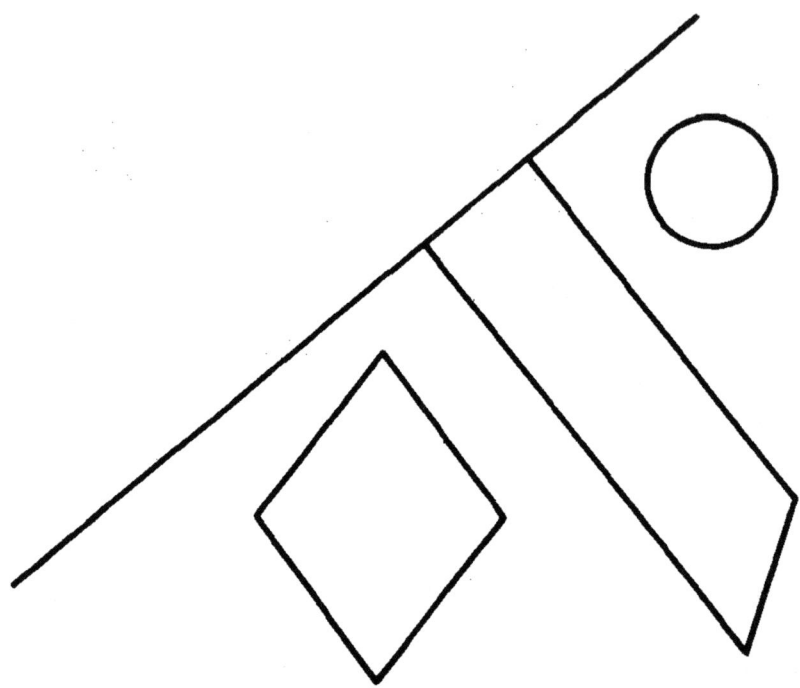

Figure 5.1. An example of a stimulus item that can be used for testing visual memory.

CONSTRUCTIONAL ABILITIES

The term *constructional abilities* refers to the ability to draw or build two- or three-dimensional objects. These require a complex combination of cortical–behavioral skills, and dysfunction in any one of the component skill areas can result in an impaired performance on a constructional task. Therefore, an impaired performance should be reported as such, and the generalist should resist the temptation to interpret the problem as a right-hemisphere lesion or a fine motor-control dysfunction. Because of the complexity of skills required for successful performance, impairment of constructional abilities may be the early signs of a progressive disorder. Also chronic alcoholics and other substance abusers will sometimes show deficits in this area, even when most other areas, particularly verbal skills, are intact. This occurs because in our culture, verbal skills are the most highly practiced and overlearned. Although the general effect of substance abuse is not skill-specific, decrements in performance will appear first in the least practiced skill areas.

Drawing to command is one method of assessing constructional abilities. Ask the patient to draw simple designs such as a circle, square, and triangle. If the patient is able to perform adequately, ask the patient to draw a more complex figure, such as a clock showing a particular time. One traditional task is to ask the patient to draw a pipe.

Next, ask the patient to copy designs that have been printed on index cards. These should include the geometric figures that the patient was earlier required to draw from command. The fact that a patient can draw from command, but cannot copy a design, is important information in determining the type of deficit present.

In addition to drawing the three simple geometrical designs, the patient can be asked to copy a figure of a Greek cross, a horizontal diamond, a three-dimensional cube, or a three-dimensional pipe. The clinician should look for and report inaccuracies, distortions, and rotations of more than 45 degrees, as these are all signs of organic impairment. Additionally, the patient may persevere in drawing the design and draw more than one copy of the same stimulus, or he may fragment the design.

A method of assessing the spatial aspects of constructional deficits is to provide designs for the patient using pencils, tongue depressors, or blocks, such as those used in Koh's Block test or the Block Design subtest of the *WAIS-III* (Wechsler, 1997). When using the pencils or tongue depressors, first, place one stick at a right angle to the edge of the table and ask the patient to replicate that design with a separate stick. Then, place a stick parallel to the edge of the table with the same command. Next, place two sticks at right angles to each other. Then, place two sticks at a right angle to a third stick. Each time, ask the patient to replicate the design. Here, the clinician should pay attention to whether or not the patient is able to reproduce the angles. Not all normal patients will be able to reproduce the designs perfectly. However, deviations of more than 25–30 degrees should be noted, and can be followed up by assessment with a short standardized instrument such as the Judgment of Line Orientation or the Visual Form Discrimination to determine the perceptual contributions.

As mentioned earlier, constructional dysfunctions can be the result of a multitude of organic etiologies. If the deficit is purely in spatial arrangement, it may the result of a right-hemisphere dysfunction. If the internal details of a reproduced design are disturbed, it may the result of a left-hemisphere dysfunction. Additionally, visual dysfunction may be the result of occipital dysfunction, deficits in visual integration may be the result of varietal dysfunction, and deficits in the direction of motor activity may be the result of frontal dysfunction. The general clinician should not try to diagnose these problems, but should refer the patient to a specialist.

HIGHER COGNITIVE FUNCTIONS

Higher cognitive functions are those activities that require integration among different skill areas, the symbolic manipulation of information, abstract problem solving, planning, and judgment. There are many different cortical–behavioral skill areas that are involved in the successful completion of these tasks. As a result, if a patient shows impairment in the previously assessed skill areas, she is likely to demonstrate impaired performance in higher cognitive functions, as well. It is also possible that patients who perform adequately in the earlier cortical–behavioral skill areas may not perform adequately in these skill areas. Especially in the early stages of a progressive dementia, the basic cognitive functions may maintain their integrity, whereas the higher order cognitive functions may begin to break down.

It is also because of the complexity of these higher order functions that impaired performance may be exhibited by individuals with metabolic disorders, viral infections, or psychiatric disorders, especially thought disorders. So far, we have strongly emphasized that the generalist clinician should not perform diagnosis using these procedures. This is of paramount importance in the case of the individual who exhibits deficits only in higher order cognitive functions. Even for the specialist, diagnosis of the individual who exhibits deficits solely in higher order functions is problematic. Cutoff scores are not always a useful index in these situations, and the interpretation of results relies on the consideration of qualitative aspects of the individual's performance.

For example, performance on higher order tasks is related to a large extent on the education and experience of the individual. This is true to a certain extent for most neuropsychological functions. However, it is less true for simple sensory functions than it is for abstraction tasks.

Although it may not represent a serious problem if an individual with a history of an eighth-grade education is unable to state how a fox and a dog are alike, if a college-educated individual cannot perform the same task, it does represent a serious problem and a probable decline in abstraction skills.

The informal assessment of higher cognitive functions includes sampling the patient's fund of knowledge, the ability of the individual to manipulate old knowledge, the level of the individual's social awareness and judgment, and abstract thinking. The informal assessment will include procedures similar to procedures used in the Information, Similarities, and Arithmetic section of the *WAIS-III*. Because the patient is likely to receive the *WAIS-III* eventually, it is not a good idea to take procedures and questions directly from the *WAIS-III* or from other standardized assessment instruments. The clinician should instead formulate her own set of similar items with different content. Examples of such similar items include the following:

Similarities

How are a bucket and a coffee mug alike? (A good response is, "They both can hold liquid"; a borderline response is, "They're both round.")

How are a bed and a couch alike? (A good response is, "They're both furniture"; a borderline response is, "They both have four legs," or "You can sleep on both of them.")

General Information

Why should people make out a will? (To avoid tax problems for beneficiaries and to make sure that your estate goes to the people you prefer.) Why are blood tests required before marriage? (To screen for disease and check for possible Rh factor incompatibilities.)

Abstract Reasoning and Interpretation of Proverbs

What does this saying mean: "Don't count your chickens before they are hatched?" (One should not count on something before it happens.) What does this saying mean: "You have to sleep in the bed you made?" (People have to face the consequences of their behavior.)

Another good way to test higher order cognitive functioning is to evaluate the ability of the person to finish a conceptual series. This task will help the clinician to obtain an informal assessment of the abstract reasoning ability of the patient. For this procedure, the clinician should prepare index cards with one series of symbols on each card. Show the series to the patient and ask what comes next.

What comes next in this series?

BDFHJ _____ (L)

11, 8, 5, _____ (2)

fire, 4, strut, 5, ox, 2, real, _____ (4)

COMPLEX FUNCTIONS

There are other complex functions that do not fit well into our schema of cognitive skill areas. These functions can be readily assessed in the MSE. One of these miscellaneous areas involves what is called left–right confusion. In this condition, the patient is unable to distinguish left from right reliably. Assessing this corticobehavioral skill is simply a matter of giving the patient verbal commands that require knowledge of left and right for their successful completion. Start with easy commands, and if the patient is able to respond correctly, move on to more complex commands. For example, start by asking the patient to point to her right eye. Then ask the patient to touch his left shoulder with his left hand. Then ask the patient to point to your left hand. Finally, ask the patient to point to your right ear with her left hand.

A rare condition associated with lesions in the left parietal lobe is known as *finger agnosia*. In this condition, the patient is unable to name the fingers of his hand. This can be assessed by asking the patient to point to your left middle finger. Show the patient one of your fingers and ask the name. Finally, blindfold the patient and lightly touch one of her fingers, asking the name of the finger.

APPLICATIONS

As discussed earlier, the MSE is best conducted in a hierarchical fashion. Mental operations are complex combinations of component skills. When this fact is kept in mind, the assessment of mental operations can be conducted more efficiently. The organization of this chapter reflects current conceptions of the hierarchical organization. It is best to start by assessing the basic levels of arousal and orientation, moving through the assessment of attention, language, memory, constructional abilities, higher order cognitive functions, and, finally, the complex functions.

At each stage, failure of the patient to perform adequately has implications for the assessment of the following areas. Extremely poor performance in an early part of the MSE may indicate that the evaluation can be safely terminated. Naturally, if a patient is unconscious, the evaluation will be short. However, there are other points at which continuing the evaluation may be unnecessary. For example, if a patient demonstrates severe deficits in receptive language skills, poor performance on later sections of the MSE may not contribute further information. This is because the poor performance is likely to be due to an inability of the subject to understand what is required of him, rather than being due to impairment in the specific skill area.

Conversely, if impairment in an early part of the MSE is only moderate, continuing the evaluation may add useful information. For example, if a patient demonstrates mild deficits in receptive language, the evaluation of constructional abilities may be conducted through the use of pantomime and example.

The flexibility of the MSE increases its efficiency in uncovering information. Because the clinician can also further assess skill areas for which the patient demonstrated problematic performance, the flexibility also increases the power of the MSE. Continued experience with the use of the MSE, coupled with more extensive readings, can help improve the ability of the clinician to use the MSE. This set of procedures should be viewed as only the beginning in learning to use the MSE to assess the possibility of organic impairment.

BRIEF EVALUATIONS

Another class of patients for whom an extended MSE is recommended are those individuals for whom the clinician suspects cognitive impairment merely on the basis of clinical presentation. Of course, this is a subjective decision, the accuracy of which depends on the level of experience of the clinician with cognitively impaired individuals. In making these decisions, the clinician may elect to complete a briefer evaluation.

Folstein, Folstein, and McHugh (1975) have presented an instrument called the Mini-Mental State Exam (MMSE) for the rapid evaluation of cognitive functioning that can be used to make decisions regarding the administration of an extended MSE. The MMSE can be given in about 10 minutes, and is appropriate for use in patients with psychiatric or psychological disorders. The MMSE provides a quick assessment of orientation to date and place (but not to time or person), of attention, delayed recall, and a few select aspects of receptive and expressive language functions. The MMSE was reported to have a 24-hour test–retest reliability coefficient of 0.88 in a sample of 22 depressed patients, a 28-day test–retest reliability coefficient of 0.98 in a sample of 23 stable impaired subjects, and an interscorer reliability coefficient of 0.83 in a sample of 19 depressed subjects. The MMSE is sensitive to age and education; therefore, Crum, Anthony, Bassett, and Folstein (1993) present norms stratified by age and education which increase the utility of this instrument in screening situations. Research in an Italian population indicated the MMSE was sensitive to the effects of education in measuring decline in cases of Alzheimer's dementia (Roselli et al., 2009).

There are two alternate items that can be used to measure attention and concentration, counting backward by 7 starting with the number 100, and spelling the word "world" backward. Lopez, Charter, Mostafavi, Nibut, and Smith (2005) reported that the two methods have roughly equivalent psychometric properties. The factor structure of the MMSE in patients with Alzheimer's dementia involves two general factors, the first including orientation, memory, attention, and construction, and the second factor including language functions (Brugnolo et al., 2009).

Although the MMSE appears to be able to identify cognitive impairment in neuropsychiatric patients, and able to differentiate cognitively impaired subjects from non-impaired subjects, it does not appear to be able to separate organically impaired subjects from schizophrenic subjects. However, a score of lower than 20 points is probably indicative of organic impairment, and patients obtaining such a score should be given an extended MSE, or else referred for more intensive evaluations. The MMSE may not be sensitive to differences between patients with dementia and patients with mild cognitive impairment (DeJager, Schrinemaekaers, Honey, & Budge, 2009), but this is understandable because it identifies impairment and not etiology.

The MMSE has been criticized for having a high rate of false negatives. In particular, the MMSE may misclassify individuals with focal impairment or the beginning signs of dementia. However, the MMSE remains the single most-used short screening device, especially in medical populations. Individual MMSE subscales including orientation to time and place, delayed recall, and attention have showed significant impairment 3 years before diagnosis of vascular dementia (Lauka, Jones, Fratiglioni, & Backman, 2004). In a different light, Starrat, Fields, and Cisewski (1992) reviewed the literature on the MMSE, and concluded that in clinical populations of older individuals, the MMSE has reasonable relations with global measures of intellectual functioning, but that the relation of MMSE scores to neuroimaging data and functional evaluations is more variable. Overall, the MMSE is best thought of as a quick procedure in which positive findings have more utility than negative findings.

Another short screening device that has generated recent interest is the Neurobehavioral Cognitive Status Examination (NCSE; Northern California Neurobehavioral Group, 1988). This instrument provides a brief evaluation of level of consciousness, orientation, attention, language, constructional ability, memory, calculations, reasoning, and judgment. In the attention, language, calculations, reasoning, and judgment areas, the subject is given a single item. If the subject fails the item, it is followed by a few more items tapping the same skill area. Although the NCSE appears to be relatively sensitive to moderate or more severe dementia, more information is needed regarding its sensitivity to different diagnostic areas.

Jacobs, Bernhard, Delgado, and Strain (1977) have proposed a quick MSE for use with medical patients. In this screen, the patient is asked questions regarding orientation to date and place (but not to person or time), questions requiring fundamental arithmetic operations, questions requiring immediate and delayed memory operations, and questions requiring the subject to supply synonyms and antonyms. There was no report of the test–retest reliability of this procedure; however, the interscorer reliability was reported to be 1.0 in an extremely limited sample of six subjects. Subjects who score less than 30 points should be suspected of organic impairment, and further evaluation is indicated.

CONCLUSIONS

The MSE is a popular tool used in both inpatient and outpatient settings. It provides a very quick evaluation of numerous areas of functioning. Whereas a clinician may choose to follow up with a longer evaluation, even if it's another screening measure, the MSE can assist in determining the necessity of a more thorough evaluation, and potentially, what cognitive domains should be the focus of the evaluation.

6 Screening Tests of Perceptual and Motor Functions

Traditionally, research conducted in neuropsychology has been directed toward the differentiation of the brain-damaged patient from all other patients. This research has focused on developing either a single test or a battery of tests that have the ability to make this discrimination. Although the comprehensive neuropsychological evaluation is more likely to encompass aspects of functional adaptation or prediction of everyday behavior, in the neuropsychological screening examination, the clinician has the responsibility of assessing unselected cases to identify areas in which additional evaluation is necessary. This generally occurs in psychiatric hospitals, rehabilitation facilities, mental health clinics, or private practice situations, in which psychological screening is routine with each patient. In these settings, examiners and clinicians usually do not choose to use a lengthy test battery because of the time and expense involved. A complete neuropsychological evaluation can routinely take 6 or more hours, and the initial evaluation can cost as much as $2400. The initial cost of purchasing the testing materials can cost as much as $4000. Many psychiatric hospitals and mental health clinics have neither the personnel nor the space to devote to such lengthy examination procedures. This is particularly true in instances in which the base rate of neurological dysfunction is low in the population being screened. In these settings, a neuropsychological screening can be used effectively and efficiently to identify those individuals whose cases would be clarified through the use of more comprehensive examinations. And in those cases, the traditional instruments used to make a binary decision of cognitively impaired versus cognitively intact still have utility.

The screening examination is not an end in itself, because the conclusions obtained are quite limited. Rather, the clinician can determine whether the possibility of neuropsychological dysfunction exists. The screening tests and batteries that will be discussed in this chapter will not be able to identify the nature of a given disorder or the primary deficits in the patient's functioning. Nor can such an examination provide a reliable aid for treatment and rehabilitation.

The clinician who uses screening devices can use one of two approaches. First, he may employ a variety of tests that are highly sensitive to brain damage in general. Second, he can use a small battery of tests that can be analyzed in much the same fashion as a larger, more comprehensive test battery. The tests in such a battery need to be selected so that each is sensitive to a different type of dysfunction, rather than the more global tests most appropriate for the first technique. All of the procedures mentioned here are more sensitive to one kind of brain damage than to another. Thus, the tests selected for a screening must complement each other, with as little redundancy as possible.

The remainder of this book, therefore, will concentrate on experimental and commercially available tests that have been shown to be sensitive to cognitive dysfunction. Finally, we will also examine ways in which effort and motivation are evaluated.

VISUAL FUNCTIONS

There are a variety of aspects of visual functioning that can be impaired by brain dysfunction. Although there are many forms of neurologic disorder that have little or no effect on visual processing, impairment in this area can be indicative of some form of central nervous system dysfunction. Therefore, the clinician may wish to include some form of screening procedure for visual functions in an evaluation. Information obtained during the clinical interview may alert the clinician to the need for including such an instrument. The patient may not always be aware of impairment in this area, and may not report it explicitly. However, reports that the patient has difficulty judging distances while driving and has demonstrated difficulty performing everyday manual functions, such as avoiding obstacles while walking or handling a coffee cup, may alert the clinician to perform a visual screening. Additionally, reports that the patient has experienced difficulty recognizing familiar faces (not just remembering names) may reflect impairment in visual processing. In testing language functions using confrontational naming, the patient may misname the object presented by naming a similar-shaped object, such as may be seen in visual stimulus errors on the Boston Naming Test (Goodglass, Kaplan, & Weintraub, 2001).

A major division in visual functions occurs between those involving verbal–symbolic material and those dealing with nonsymbolic stimuli. Other stimulus dimensions that may highlight different aspects of visual perception are the degree to which the stimulus is structured, the amount of remote and new memory involved in the task, spatial relationships, and the presence of interfering information. We will start with tests for the more basic functions, such as simple perception and recognition, and progress to higher order tasks, such as visual–spatial relationships.

Color Perception

Although formal tests of color perception are not typically used in evaluations conducted by psychologists, screening for color perception can serve a dual purpose in the assessment of patients in whom brain dysfunction is suspected, or identify individuals with color blindness who cannot perform tasks requiring accurate color recognition (such as the Wisconsin Card Sorting test [Heaton, 1999] or Stroop Color Word Test [Golden, 1978]).

Two popular tests of color perception are the Ishihara (1983) and the Dvorine (1953) screening tests. Both of these tests are venerable procedures that can also be found in general physicians' offices, as well as optometrists' and ophthalmologists' offices. Psychologists may remember these tests from their undergraduate introductory texts. Each test requires that the patient view a card printed with different colored dots that form recognizable figures against a background of contrasting colored dots. All of the dots are matched for color saturation. Individuals with defective color perception will be unable to see the stimulus figure against the background. In contrast, those patients with intact color vision and color agnosia will be able to make the discriminations necessary, but may not be able to differentiate between a red ball and a blue ball.

The Color Perception Battery (DeRenzi & Spinnler, 1967) includes the Ishihara plates, as well as tests of color matching, pointing to color, color drawing, color naming, and memory for colors. The purpose of this instrument is the discrimination of those individuals whose difficulty arises from purely perceptual deficits from those with a language component (aphasia), from those patients with other forms of the loss of knowledge about object colors.

VISUAL RECOGNITION

Assessment of visual processing can be technically difficult (Beaumont & Davidoff, 1992). Visual processing deficits can cover numerous dimensions, including location, size, brightness, contrast, movement, color, complexity, and sequence. In most instances, the general clinician will have neither the specialized training nor the equipment required to perform this type of assessment. However inadequate it may be methodologically, the clinician will typically be limited to a simple confrontational assessment of the visual fields, leaving detailed examinations to others—specially trained neuropsychologists (not all neuropsychologists have been adequately trained for this) and others who can perform psychophysical assessments.

A commonly used test that can be used to assess visual recognition is the *Peabody Picture Vocabulary Test-IV* (*PPVT-IV*; Dunn & Dunn, 2007). The *PPVT* was designed primarily to assess an individual's receptive vocabulary skills. It is an effective tool for assessing aspects of both aphasia and perceptual functions. In the standard administration of the test, the patient is shown a series of pages, each of which has four pictures on it. The patient is required to indicate, either verbally or nonverbally, which of the four pictures on a given page best shows a word spoken by the examiner. A raw score is then calculated in terms of the total number of correct responses, which can then be converted into a number of standard or derived scores based on a large normative database. This procedure can give the clinician a fairly good idea as to whether a picture recognition deficit exists, from which the presence of possible brain dysfunction can be inferred. Although this test can be used to assess visual functions, it is important to rule out language dysfunction. Of course, if there is impaired performance when this test is used for screening purposes, it may be helpful to refer the patient for more comprehensive neuropsychological evaluation, regardless of the underlying dysfunction.

Face Recognition

Warrington and James (1967) demonstrated a difference between the inability to recognize familiar faces (prosopagnosia) and impaired recognition of unfamiliar faces. Therefore, facial recognition tests can be divided into those that involve a memory component and those that do not. Tests of familiar facial recognition require a memory component, and generally use the faces of popular figures and well-known historical figures; the memory element is one of the difficulties with this form of test. If a patient performs poorly on such a test, it is quite difficult to determine whether the primary problem involves perceptual recognition or visual memory.

In order to evaluate the ability to recognize faces without involving memory, Benton et al. (1994) developed the Test of Facial Recognition. In this test, the patient is asked to match photographs of an unknown person with either identical photographs, photographs taken from the side, or photographs taken under different lighting conditions. A patient with problems in facial recognition usually will have right-hemisphere dysfunction. Neither visual field defects nor the presence of aphasia will affect visual recognition scores (Lezak, Howieson, & Loring, 2004); however, facial recognition deficits do tend to occur with spatial agnosia and dyslexia, as well as with dysgraphias (problems with writing) that involve spatial disturbance (Tzavaras, Hecaen, & Le Bras, 1970).

Figure and Design Recognition

Simple Recognition

Perceptual recognition of meaningless designs is generally tested by having the subject draw a variety of designs from memory or from model figures. When a patient's design reproductions contain the essential elements of the original from which they were copied and preserve the proper interrelationships with general accuracy, the patient's perception has been adequately demonstrated (Lezak et al., 2004). The capacity to recognize meaningful information can be rapidly assessed using the *Wechsler Adult Intelligence Scale* (*WAIS-IV*; Wechsler, 2008) Picture Completion subtest.

There are a number of other techniques that can be used to assess simple perceptual recognition. A very low-level test of visual recognition can be found in the Discrimination of Forms subtest of the *Stanford-Binet* (Roid, 2003). The patient is shown 10 line drawings of common geometric figures (such as a square, circle, etc.), one at a time, and asked to point out the matching figure on a card on which all 10 figures are displayed. The first 12 items of Raven's Progressive Matrices (Raven, 1960) can also be used as a test of simple recognition ability (Knehr, 1965).

There are also several devices that have been developed to ascertain intact perceptual closure, including the Street Completion Test (Street, 1931), the Mooney Closure Test (Mooney & Ferguson, 1951), and the Gestalt Completion Test (Ekstrom, French, Harman, & Dermen, 1976). Although these tests can discriminate patients from controls, the tests are not well correlated with each other in normal subjects. Beaumont and Davidoff (1992) report that the Gollin Incomplete Figures (Gollin, 1960) is a useful instrument to assess recognition. The test comprises 20 sets of stimuli, each set of which is a progressively more complete representation of an object. The test assesses the ability to extract perceptual features (Warrington & Rabin, 1970).

COMPLEX VISUAL FUNCTIONS—TESTS OF SPATIAL ABILITIES

Tests of complex visual abilities have long been popular as single tests of brain injury. This popularity appears to be based on the known representation of complex spatial functions in both cerebral hemispheres (Golden, 1981).

Bender Visual–Motor Gestalt

The Bender Visual–Motor Gestalt Test has a long history of being used for assessing visual processing. In the past, clinicians had a tendency to use the Bender, and only the Bender, to identify possible cortical dysfunction. This approach should be avoided, because the Bender Visual–Motor Gestalt has not been shown effectively to perform this exclusive function. The danger of this use lies in the Bender's high rate of false negative findings related to cortical dysfunction. However, it can be used as a quick screening procedure to examine spatial abilities.

In using the Bender, the clinician asks the patient to copy nine geometric figures and patterns on a blank sheet of paper. The drawings are then evaluated by one of several scoring systems that have been developed over the years. Each of these scoring systems has attempted to identify qualitative signs indicating brain damage. In some cases, variations of these scoring approaches also attempt to identify emotional disorders. The most popular of these scoring systems include those presented by Bender (1938), Hain (1964), Hutt (1969), and Pascal and Suttell (1951).

Investigators who have used these scoring systems have reported up to 70% accuracy in identifying brain-injured individuals, and a hit rate of 90% in identifying normal subjects (e.g., Brilliant & Gynther, 1963; Levine & Feirstein, 1972; Tymchuk, 1974). However, there have been a number of other studies using the Bender that have reported essentially negative results, particularly in those situations in which the differentiation between brain-damaged and psychiatric patients was required (Johnson, Hellkamp, & Lottman, 1971; Mosher & Smith, 1965; Watson, 1968). Several major review articles have criticized the Bender Visual–Motor Gestalt Test for its unreliability and inability to discriminate in psychiatric populations. Studies using the Bender have also received a good deal of criticism for not using control subjects (Billingslea, 1963; Canter, 1966; Tolor & Schulberg, 1963). The results of this research indicate that the use of the Bender by itself allows far too wide a margin for error in clinical work. A poor score on the Bender may indeed indicate problems for a client; however, it does not specify the nature of the patient's problems. Similarly, and perhaps more importantly, a good score on the Bender does not rule out the possibility of the presence of brain damage. The Bender does its job well as a visual–perceptual screening device when it is used in conjunction with other tests. It should never be used as the sole index of brain damage when screening a patient for the presence of cortical dysfunction.

Benton Visual Retention Test

The Benton Visual Retention Test (BVRT) consists of three alternate but equivalent versions that may be administered under differing conditions

(Benton, 1974; Sivan, 1991). The conditions include simple copying and copying from memory after a delay (no delay and 15-second delay). Each version of the test consists of 10 cards with more than one figure in the horizontal plane. The copy condition of the test is sensitive to disruptions in visual–spatial processing.

As its name implies, the BVRT is actually intended to assess visual memory. However, its utility as a screening device can be enhanced by asking the subject to simply copy the designs or to match the target stimuli with the correct alternative among those provided by the examiner.

Each version of the test is scored for both the number of correct designs and the number of errors. Six types of errors are possible: omissions, distortions, perseverations, rotations, misplacements (in the relative positioning of one figure to the others), and errors in size. Therefore, it is common to have more than one error per card. Both the number correct and the error score norms for Administration A (the most frequently used administration consisting of a 10-second exposure and then immediate copying from memory) take into account intelligence level and age. A raw score of below 4 indicates impaired functioning, regardless of age and estimated intelligence. More than nine total errors suggests impaired performance as well.

Interpretation is conducted by reference to a set of norms stratified by age and level of intellectual functioning in order to determine whether either the number correct or number of errors falls into the impaired range. Benton (1974) considers a score of 2 points below the number of expected correct responses to "raise the question of impairment," whereas a score that is four or more points below the expected score is viewed as a "strong indication" of impairment. Error scores are dealt with in a similar fashion. A patient whose error score exceeds the expected score, based on age and intelligence, by 3 or more points can be suspected of being impaired, and an error score exceeding the expected level by 5 or more points is considered a "strong indication" of brain dysfunction. Similar scoring criteria and methods are used for the other versions of the BVRT.

The manual also provides definitions of different error types. These error types include rotation, distortion, perseveration, substitution, and omission. However, there is little empirical support for the interpretation of these error types. Therefore, interpretation is conducted on the basis of theory. The BVRT is able to discriminate groups of patients with brain damage from groups with psychiatric disorders. It is not accurate enough, however, to be used singly for individual diagnostic decisions (Watson, 1968). As with other tests of visual functioning, patients with right-hemisphere lesions tend to perform more poorly than do patients with left-sided brain damage, and patients with posterior brain damage do more poorly than patients with anterior brain damage. These statements reflect only statistical associations, and are not hard-and-fast rules for diagnosis from BVRT results. The BVRT-R (Sivan, 1991) features updated and expanded normative data, as well as a reasonably detailed review of research conducted with the test. Of note is the vastly improved format of the response record, which makes recording and scoring of the test a good deal easier than was the case previously. Also, the test publisher has included a scoring template that assists in the scoring of the more detailed aspects of the individual reproductions.

Of particular interest to clinicians performing screening operations, Steck (2005) has developed a set of alternate procedures using these stimuli. The original stimuli from all of the alternate versions of the BVRT were combined into two tests with 20 items each. The items are then ordered in such a way that the test could be discontinued after four consecutive failures. Rasch model analysis (item-response theory model) indicated adequate diagnostic utility when that discontinue rule was used.

Rey-Osterrieth Complex Figure Test

A "complex figure" was devised by Rey (1941) and standardized by Osterrieth (1944). Osterrieth also obtained normative data from the performance of 230 normal children, with ages ranging from 4 to 15, and 60 adults in the 16–60 age range. He also gathered data from a small group of adults (43) with mixed brain damage. Since that time, other complex figure tests have been developed. They all have essentially the same procedures and scoring techniques. The basic procedure includes two blank sheets of paper and multiple colored pencils. The patient is first asked to copy a complex figure, which has been placed so that its length runs along the patient's horizontal plane. The examiner watches the performance closely. Each time a section of the figure is completed, a different-colored pencil is handed to the patient, and the order of the colors is recorded. Time needed to complete the figure is noted, and both the figure and drawing are removed from the patient's field of vision. After 3 minutes, the subject is given a second sheet of paper and is asked to draw the design from memory. The time to complete the drawing is recorded, as is whether the patient follows the same procedural approach on the second drawing as on the first. Normative data are used to determine the correct score and the patient's performance. Some clinicians prefer to use the Rey-Osterrieth over the Bender or the BVRT because it also allows an assessment of memory and execution function.

Block Design and Other Construction Tests

Block design tests require the patient to reproduce a pattern, usually using multicolored blocks. Most psychologists are familiar with the Block Design subtest of the Wechsler Intelligence Scales (Wechsler, 1945). The patient is shown a picture of a red-and-white design and asked to replicate that design using either two, four, or nine red-and-white blocks. The blocks have two sides that are completely white, two sides that are completely red, and two sides that are half red and half white, split along the diagonal. This test is most sensitive to right-hemisphere lesions (McFie, 1975). However, left-hemisphere injuries, especially those in the parietal lobe (McFie, 1960) or those involving more severe damage, may also affect performance on this test. Golden (1977) demonstrated that the test is effective in identifying over 80% of patients with either right-hemisphere or diffuse dysfunction. It is important to recognize that the procedures discussed in this section are tests of construction, a construct that requires more than just intact visual processing. Certainly, visual processing deficits can produce impaired performance on construction tasks, but so can visual motor integration impairment and executive dysfunction. If the screening clinician is uncertain about the reason for deficient performance on construction tasks, he can produce accurate and inaccurate models of the stimuli and ask the patient to match the correct designs or identify whether the models produced by the clinician are accurate or inaccurate.

Raven's Progressive Matrices

This test was originally designed as a culture-free measure of intelligence (Raven, 1960). Although subsequent research has found that the test

Chapter 6 Tests of Perceptual and Motor Functions 113

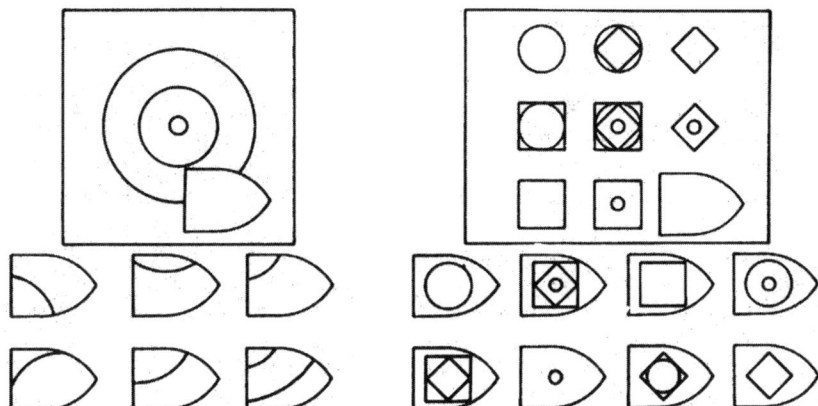

Figure 6.1. Examples of the Raven's Progressive Matrices Test.

did not meet this goal, it does appear to offer a measure of nonverbal reasoning. The test is quite easy to administer and can be given with little formal training. There are no time limits, and the test generally takes from 40 minutes to 1 hour. It consists of 60 items grouped into 5 series, plus 2 sample items. Each item contains a pattern problem with one part missing and from four to eight pictured inserts, one of which contains the correct pattern (see Figure 6.1). The subject points to the pattern piece he feels will complete the larger pattern. Alternatively, the patient can write the response on an answer sheet. There is also a version for children and adults of low intellectual level—the Coloured Progressive Matrices—as well as a computerized version.

Clock Drawing

The Clock Drawing Test is a simple, quick clinical screening for visual spatial and constructional deficits. It has been used as a part of a standard brief mental status examination (MSE) in neurology for some time (e.g., Strub & Black, 1977). The test requires a sheet of paper and a pencil. The patient is told to draw the face of a clock with all the numbers on it and to make it large. Once the patient has completed her drawing, she is told to draw the hands at 20 minutes to 4. The instructions can be repeated or paraphrased as needed, but no other help should be offered.

The task is scored as follows: A 10-point scoring system is used. A score of 10 is awarded if it is a normal drawing with the numbers and hands in roughly the correct positions. The hour hand should be distinctly different from the minute hand and approaching 4 o'clock. A score of 9 is received if there are slight errors in the placement of the hands (not exactly on the 8 and 4, but not on one of the adjoining numbers) or one missing number from the face of the clock. Eight points are given with more noticeable errors in the placement of the hour and minute hand (off by one number), or if the number spacing shows a gap. A score of 7 is given if the hands are placed significantly off the mark (more than one number), or there is inappropriate spacing of the numbers (all numbers on one side of the clock). Six points are scored with inappropriate use of the clock hands (use of a digital display or circling of the numbers despite repeated instructions, or the crowding of numbers at one end of the clock or a reversal of numbers). The patient receives a score of 5 when there is a perseverative or otherwise inappropriate arrangement (e.g., numbers indicated by dots). Also this score is given if the hands are represented, but do not clearly point at a number. Four points are received when numbers are absent, written outside of the clock, if they are distorted in sequence, or if the hands are not clearly represented. A score of 3 points is given when numbers and face are no longer connected in the drawing or the hands are not recognizably present. A score of 2 is given when the drawing reveals some evidence that the instructions were understood, but the representation of the clock is vague, at best. Typically, there is an inappropriate spatial arrangement of numbers. Finally, a score of 1 point is attained when there is no attempt or the attempt is not recognizable.

Currently available norms suggest that scores of 7–10 represent normal functioning (Sunderland et al., 1989; Wolf-Klein, Silverstone, Levy, & Brod, 1989). A score of 6 is thought to be borderline impaired. Scores of 5 or less are rare in normal functioning individuals. Berger, Frolich, Weber, and Pantel (2008) provide support for the utility of asking the patient to draw the hands of the clock to represent a particular time. Peters and Pinto (2008) suggest that the Clock Drawing Test may not only identify current impairment, but may also predict future decline. Kim, Lee, Choi, Sohn, and Lee (2009) provide data to suggest that performance on the Clock Drawing Test is associated with white matter hyperintensity and medial temporal lobe atrophy.

Trail Making Test

The Trail Making Test (Army Individual Test, 1944) is a popular test of visual–conceptual and visuomotor tracking. Because it requires attention, it can be affected by a variety of different forms of brain damage (Reitan, 1958). It is given in two parts, A and B (see Figure 6.2). The patient is asked to draw lines connecting consecutively numbered circles on one page (Part A), and then is asked to connect the same number of consecutively numbered and lettered circles on another page by alternating between letters and numbers (Part B). The examiner records both the time required and the number of errors made, as well as pointing out the errors to the patient so they can be corrected. The time this takes is reflected in the total time required to complete each section. These procedures are simple, short, and sensitive, although not specific. The Trail Making Test, Part B, is itself one of the most sensitive to a wide variety of neurocognitive impairments.

As is the case for all test performances scored on speed alone, it must be remembered that allowances need to be made for normal aging, because psychomotor speed tends to decrease with age. The Trail Making Test is no exception to this, as performance time has been found to decrease with each succeeding decade (Davies, 1968). Table 6.1 demonstrates this trend in normal control subjects.

In general, cutoff scores are used for determining whether performance is impaired on the Trail Making Test. For younger individuals, aged 20–39, normal performance time on Part A should be 50 seconds or less, and 79 seconds or less for Part B. The combined time to complete both Parts A and B should be less than 110 seconds. However, when these cutoff criteria are applied to normal individuals in their 70s the scores misclassify an average of 91% as being brain damaged. Therefore, it is important to account for the age of the patient being tested and for the distributions of scores achieved by normal older subjects. More recent research has indicated that the Trail Making Test is sensitive to differences among normal healthy older subjects, subjects with mild cognitive impairment, and subjects with dementia (Ashendorf et al., 2008), especially when the number of errors is taken into account. These researchers found that the presence of an error on Trail Making Test B was less sensitive to aging effects than the time score, and that using both (requiring time over the cutoff and the presence of one or more errors) increased the accuracy in classifying older subjects as either healthy or diagnosed with dementia.

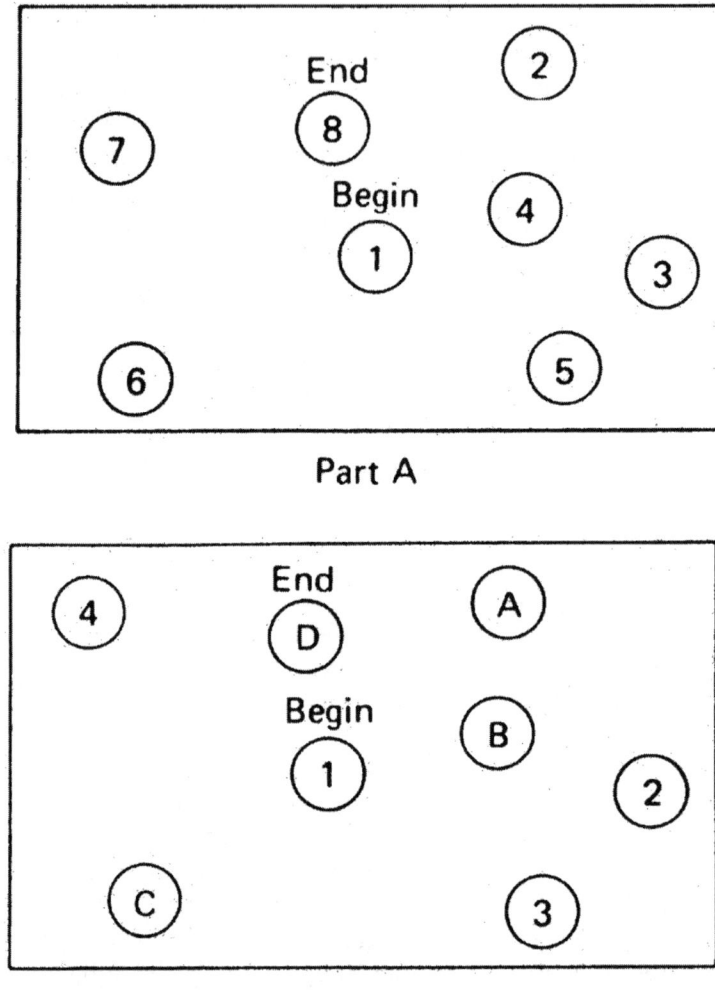

Figure 6.2. Practice samples of the Trail Making Test.

When the time taken to complete Part A is relatively far less than that needed to complete Part B, it is likely that the patient has difficulty in complex conceptual tracking or sequencing. Slow performance at any age on one or both parts of the test points to the likelihood of brain damage, but does not indicate whether the problem is one of

Table 6.1

TRAIL MAKING TEST SCORES[a] FOR CONTROL SUBJECTS

AGE	20–39 (N = 180)		40–49 (N = 90)		50–59 (N = 90)		60–69 (N = 90)		70–79 (N = 90)	
PART	A	B	A	B	A	B	A	B	A	B
PERCENTILE										
90	21	45	22	49	25	55	29	64	38	79
75	26	55	28	57	29	75	35	89	54	132
50	32	69	34	78	38	98	48	119	80	196
25	42	94	45	100	49	135	67	172	105	292
10	50	129	59	151	67	177	104	282	168	450

[a]Scores are in seconds.
Note: From Davies, A. (1968). The influence of age on Trail Making Test performance. *Journal of Clinical Psychology, 24.* Adapted by permission.

motor slowing, poor coordination, visual scanning difficulties, poor motivation, or conceptual confusion (Lezak et al., 2004).

AUDITORY FUNCTIONS

Auditory functions involve both verbal and nonverbal aspects (Milner, 1962). Auditory functions can be noticeably impaired, and may be a frequent reason for referral for evaluation. Because verbal interaction is an important component of everyday life, much attention has been focused on developing tests for assessing verbal auditory functions. However, there has been less attention paid to developing tests that assess nonverbal auditory functions.

Every comprehensive neuropsychological evaluation provides some opportunity to evaluate the auditory perception of verbal material. This is also the case for a neuropsychological screening. When the examiner orally presents problems of judgment and reasoning, learning, and memory, the opportunity also arises to conduct an informal assessment of the patient's auditory acuity and comprehension, as well as of processing capacity. Significant deficits in the perception and comprehension of speech can become readily apparent quite rapidly during the course of administering most psychological tests.

If a few tasks with simple instructions requiring only motor responses or one or two word answers are given, however, subtle problems with auditory processing may be missed. These include difficulty in processing or retaining lengthy messages, although responses to single words or phrases may be accurate; inability to handle spoken numbers without a concomitant impairment in processing other forms of speech; or an inability to process information at high levels in the auditory system when the ability to repeat them accurately remains intact. In the absence of a primary hearing disorder, any impairment in the individual's capacity to recognize or effectively process speech typically indicates a lesion in the dominant cerebral hemisphere (Milner, 1962).

When impairment in auditory processing is suspected, the clinician can couple an auditorily presented test with a similar task presented visually. This enables the clinician to compare the functioning of both perceptual systems under similar conditions. If the patient demonstrates a consistent tendency to perform better under one of the two conditions, the possibility of neurological impairment of the less-efficient perceptual system exists. Pairs of tests can be readily found or developed for most verbal tests at most levels of difficulty. For instance, a series of tasks requiring both written and mental computations can be used.

TACTILE FUNCTIONS

The assessment of tactile perception, or the ability to be aware of touch perception, involves simple recognition or discrimination problems. For example, the patient may be asked to simply state whether tactile stimulation has occurred or where the stimulation was localized. However, there are some formal measures of tactile perception presented in the text that follows.

Tactile Recognition and Discrimination Tests

The detailed examination for finger agnosia (Kinsbourne & Warrington, 1962) includes three tactile tests that require no elaborate equipment. The patient is asked to close his eyes (alternatively, the patient can be blindfolded) and place the hands, palms down, on the working surface for all of these tests. These tests should be given first with the patient's eyes open to ensure that the tasks are understood. In the *In-between Test*, the examiner touches two fingers simultaneously, having instructed the patient to tell the number of fingers in between the two that are touched. The *Two-Point Finger Test* requires that the examiner touch two places on the same or different fingers; the patient is asked to tell whether one or two fingers were touched. In the *Match Box Test*, the examiner slips a small match box between two of the patient's fingers or touches the sides of two different fingers with two match boxes. The patient is required to tell which fingers were touched. Of these three tests, the In-Between Test has consistently been found to be the most clinically useful (Lezak et al., 2004). Patients with finger agnosia consistently had difficulty differentiating their fingers or relating one to another. Control subjects with some form of cortical dysfunction but no evidence of finger agnosia performed these tests without error.

Benton, Hamsher, Varney, and Spreen (1983) have described a version of this procedure that consists of 60 items broken into three sections: (a) with the hand visible, localization of single fingers touched by the examiner with the pointed end of a pencil (10 trials on each hand); (b) with the hand hidden from view, localization of single fingers touched by the examiner (10 trials on each hand); (c) with the hand hidden from view, localization of fingers touched simultaneously by the examiner (10 trials on each hand). The mode of response is left to the patient. She can name the touched fingers, point to them on an outline drawing of the stimulated hand, or call out their numbers. Throughout the test, the patient's hands rest on the table with the palms up, and fingers extended and separated slightly. In those individuals with a spastic movement disorder in which the hand and fingers cannot be positioned to allow for a valid assessment, finger-localization testing is limited to the unaffected hand. Several performance patterns have been reported using this approach (Benton et al., 1983). *Normal performance* is reflected by a score of 51–60 (single-hand score of 25–30, with right–left difference of 0–3 points). *Borderline normal* performance results from a total score of 49–51 (one single-hand score of 26–27 and one single-hand score of 23–24, with right–left difference of 0–3 points). *Bilateral symmetric impairment* is present when single-hand scores are less than 26, with right–left differences of 0–3 points. Generally, when the right–left score is greater than 4 points, the greatest defect is reflected by the hand with the poorest performance.

Object recognition without the aid of vision (stereognosis) is commonly performed in a standard neurological examination. The patient is required to recognize by touch common objects such as a coin, pencil, key, and so forth, while his/her eyes are closed. Procedures occur for each hand separately. Size and texture discrimination can be easily assessed. It has been reported that adults with no evidence of brain injury can perform tactile recognition and discrimination tests with total accuracy. A single error, or even evidence of hesitancy, is a strong suggestion that this function is impaired, and is typically associated with lesions on the contralateral hemisphere (Weinstein, 1964).

Reitan-Klove Sensory Perceptual Examination

This test combines much of the tactile perceptual examination techniques discussed previously into a single package, which is comparatively easy for an experienced clinician to administer. However, it is important that the clinician receive some training in the administration of this series of tests; they can easily be administered improperly, yielding useless findings. Proper administration is essential for useful and interpretable results.

This test was developed by Reitan and Klove (Reitan, n.d.), and draws on a long history of similar tests used in neurology. The first part of the test evaluates the presence of sensory suppressions, using double simultaneous stimulation in the tactile, auditory, and visual modalities. Tests for the perception of single stimulation are included, because suppressions cannot be scored unless it is clear that the patient is able to perceive unilateral stimulation. The patient is asked to close her eyes and place her hands on the table. The examiner then proceeds randomly to touch either one of the patient's hands, either side of the patient's face, both hands, both sides of the face, or one hand and the opposite side of the face. It is important that bilateral stimulation be done simultaneously and with equal pressure, or else the patient will be receiving two unilateral stimuli, thus defeating the purpose of the examination. There should be no discernible pattern to the touching, and each hand, as well as each side of the face, should receive an equal number of both unilateral and simultaneous stimulations. The test is scored in terms of errors.

To assess the presence of auditory perception deficits, the examiner stands behind the patient and rubs his fingers together slightly behind, but close to, the patient's ears. The clinician then asks the patient to tell on which side the noise was made—right, left, or both at once. The examiner should be careful to make the stimulus noise just audible to the patient and to assess unilateral, as well as bilateral, simultaneous perceptual functioning. As above, total errors are scored.

Assessment for visual suppression is done in a similar manner. The examiner sits about 3 feet away from the front of the patient and asks the patient to fixate on the examiner's nose. The examiner's hands are then held at about an arm's length away from the examiner's body, and one or two fingers are moved slightly. The patient is then asked on which side the movement occurred—left or right. Bilateral presentations also occur. The examiner again should be sure to give the patient an equal number of unilateral and double simultaneous stimulations. The upper, middle, and lower portions of the patient's visual fields should be assessed in this manner.

If no primary sensory deficit is in evidence, as indicated by correct identification of unilateral stimulations, even one error in double simultaneous stimulation can be indicative of cerebral dysfunction. The clinician must be certain that the suppression error was a valid suppression and not the result of a temporary lapse in the patient's attention. Genuine suppressions are quite rare, but are almost always indicative of brain injury.

MANUAL MOTOR FUNCTIONING

It is important to include a measure or measures of manual motor control, speed, and dexterity in a neuropsychological screening battery. Examination of these areas may assist in identifying organic impairment. Many of these tests can be administered quickly with limited instructions.

Finger Tapping Test

The Finger Tapping Test (Reitan & Davison, 1974), which was originally called the Finger Oscillation Test by Halstead (1947), is another procedure that had a prior history as a stand-alone test and was then incorporated into the Halstead-Reitan battery. The patient is asked to tap a device that records the number of taps. Each hand performs five 10-second trials, with brief rest periods interspersed between trials. The scores for each hand are then averaged across the five trials. Normal right-handed individuals average 50 taps per 10-second trial for their dominant hand and 45 taps for the nondominant hand. As with other motor tasks, age and sex will affect expected performance levels. The presence of cortical damage tends to have a slowing effect on the finger-tapping rate. Lateralized lesions may result in a marked slowing of the tapping rate of the hand contralateral to the lesion. However, such effects do not appear with enough frequency or consistency to warrant the use of this test as a screening for lateralized damage. Diffuse damage will lead to a generalized slowing of the tapping rate of both hands. In general, the clinician can expect to see about a 10% difference in the tapping rates of the two hands, with the dominant hand being faster.

Grip Strength

As we have noted, examining the patient's level of performance and comparing performance on both sides of the body can be useful in determining the integrity of brain functioning. Clinicians have realized that intensity or strength of voluntary motor activity can also be a reliable indicator of brain functions. Many neuropsychologists use some strength-of-grip measure in comprehensive evaluations. A measure of grip strength can also be used in a screening evaluation.

Reitan and Davison (1974) established the hand dynamometer as having clinical value for such purposes. Testing the strength of a patient's grip requires the use of a dynamometer, which can be adjusted to the size of the patient's hands. The patient is asked to extend his preferred hand downward and is then instructed to squeeze as hard as possible. Two trials are given to each hand in alternating fashion. The final score for each hand is the average of the two trials. The dominant-hand result should be 10% greater than that of the nondominant hand.

Clinicians who may wish to consider using the Grip Strength Test should be warned that although the test is a reasonably good indicator of brain dysfunction in a number of instances, it cannot be used as the sole measure; it is not accurate enough to do so.

The Purdue Pegboard Test

The Purdue Pegboard Test examines manual dexterity and is sensitive to lateralized lesions (Costa, Vaughan, Levita, & Farber, 1963). In this task, the patient places pegs in holes on a board arranged in lines first with his dominant hand, then his nondominant hand, and then both hands simultaneously. The total amount of pegs that are placed within the 30 seconds is the score for each condition. Cortical dysfunction may decrease scores generally, and unilaterally low scores may reflect contralateral brain damage. Extensive normative data is provided in Strauss, Sherman, and Spreen (2006) for children as young as 5 years old.

Because the total testing time, including instructions and practice, rarely exceeds 5 minutes, the Purdue Pegboard can be a highly efficient method of screening for cortical dysfunction and detecting a possible lesion. Because it is not only brief, but also unlikely to unduly fatigue a patient, it can be readily included in most screening batteries; however, the test's size and weight may place limits on its portability in some situations.

CONCLUSIONS

Examining for perceptual and motor impairment is challenging, given the numerous deficits that may be present. Difficulties range from visual-based or other sensory impairments to ataxia. It is easy to overlook perceptual deficits, and may not be diagnosed unless other cognitive skills, such as memory, are affected. Whereas overt motor difficulties, such as tremors and gait problems, are easy to diagnose, the challenge of the clinician is to determine whether it is merely a symptom of an underlying disorder, as is often the case. Understanding relatively quick measures used to diagnose these skills may assist the clinician in determining the necessity of referring to a neurologist or other specialist for further evaluation.

7 Screening Tests for Verbal Functions

TESTS FOR APHASIA

Aphasia is the acquired inability to demonstrate particular aspects of language. It can either be receptive or expressive in nature. Therefore, almost any test which uses verbal instructions or oral requests for information is sensitive to the presence of aphasia. Specific tests for aphasia, however, differ from other verbal assessment devices, in that they focus on language-based skills and abilities. Such tests have been designed to elicit samples of an individual's behavior in each of the various language modalities of listening, speaking, reading, writing, and gesturing. An important consideration in selecting screening instruments for aphasia is to determine which language skills are of interest to the clinician. Subsequently, knowledge of which measures can be used both quickly and efficiently is necessary.

Screening tests assessing aphasia are not designed to replace a careful examination of language functions afforded by comprehensive language assessment batteries, as they do not provide fine discrimination (Eisenson, 1973; Rabin, Barr, & Burton, 2005). There are a variety of thorough language assessments available to do so (Spreen & Risser, 2003). Rather, screening measures can signal the presence of a disorder, and may even identify specific characteristics. Screening measures can be easily administered and interpreted by clinicians who are not experts of the different aphasias, because they do not require technical knowledge of speech pathology for acceptable administration or interpretation.

General Aphasia Screening Instruments

The Aphasia Screening Test (AST) or one of its many variations has been incorporated into many organized neuropsychological test batteries. As originally developed, Halstead and Wepman's (1949) AST has 51 items that covers all aspects of language skills. It typically requires less than 30 minutes to complete. The purpose of the test is to identify the presence of a communication problem with a secondary goal of understanding the nature of the aphasia. The AST has no rigid scoring standards, and errors are coded into a profile that can provide a description of the pattern of language disabilities. The test is not designed to assess performance on the basis of severity of the problem. However, the more areas involved, and possibly the higher frequency of an involved area, suggests a greater severity of dysfunction.

Reitan included the AST in the Halstead-Reitan Neuropsychological Test Battery, which is described elsewhere. He reduced the original test to 32 items, but still handled the data in a descriptive fashion, in much the same manner as originally intended (Reitan & Wolfson, 1985). This shortened version of the AST is the one most commonly used and is readily available. Table 7.1 and Figure 7.1 present the tasks in the AST as well as the organization of the items.

A second revision of the AST appeared in Russell, Neuringer, and Goldstein's (1970) amplification of the Halstead-Reitan Test Battery. This version of the original Halstead and Wepman test is called the "Aphasia Examination" and contains 37 items. It is basically the same as the Reitan revision, with the addition of four simple arithmetic problems and the task of naming a key. A very short version of the AST was developed by Heimburger and Reitan in 1961 and consists of four tasks: copying a square, Greek cross, and triangle without lifting the pencil from the paper; naming each copied figure; spelling each name; and repeating, explaining, and writing the phrase, "He shouted the warning."

Other brief aphasia screening tests have recently been developed and validated with the goal of being effective and efficient. As noted

Table 7.1

MODIFIED HALSTEAD-WEPMAN AST ITEMS

TASK	INSTRUCTIONS TO PATIENT
1. Copy SQUARE (A)	FIRST, DRAW THIS ON YOUR PAPER (point to square, item A). I WANT YOU TO DO IT WITHOUT LIFTING YOUR PENCIL FROM THE PAPER. TRY TO MAKE IT ABOUT THE SAME SIZE (elaborate as necessary). If patient is concerned about making a heavy or double line, note that only a reproduction of the shape is necessary. If patient encounters difficulty in shape reproduction, encourage patient to do his or her best. If the task is not accomplished reasonably well on the first attempt, ask patient to try again.
2. Name SQUARE	WHAT IS THAT SHAPE CALLED?
3. Spell SQUARE	WOULD YOU SPELL THAT WORD FOR ME?
4. Copy CROSS (B)	DRAW THIS ON YOUR PAPER (point to cross). GO AROUND THE OUTSIDE LIKE THIS UNTIL YOU GET BACK WHERE YOU STARTED (examiner draws a finger line around the edge of the figure). MAKE IT ABOUT THE SAME SIZE. Additional instructions are given in the same manner as those used for the square as needed.
5. Name CROSS	WHAT IS THAT SHAPE CALLED?
6. Spell CROSS	WOULD YOU SPELL THAT WORD FOR ME?
7. Copy TRIANGLE (C)	Similar to instructions for 1 and 4.
8. Name TRIANGLE	WHAT IS THAT SHAPE CALLED?
9. Spell TRIANGLE	WOULD YOU SPELL THAT WORD FOR ME?
10. Name BABY (D)	WHAT IS THIS? (Show item D).
11. Write CLOCK (E)	NOW I AM GOING TO SHOW YOU ANOTHER PICTURE, BUT DO NOT TELL ME THE NAME OF IT. DON'T SAY ANYTHING OUT LOUD. JUST WRITE THE NAME OF THE PICTURE ON THE PAPER (show item E).
12. Name FORK (F)	WHAT IS THIS? (show item F).
13. Read 7 SIX 2 (G)	I WANT YOU TO READ THIS (show item G). If patient has difficulty, attempt to determine whether any of the stimulus figures can be read.

Table 7.1 *(continued)*

14. Read M G W (H)	READ THIS (show item H).
15. Reading I (I)	READ THIS (show item I).
16. Reading II (J)	TRY TO READ THIS (show item J).
17. Repeat TRIANGLE	NOW I AM GOING TO SAY SOME WORDS. I WANT YOU TO LISTEN CAREFULLY AND SAY THEM AS CAREFULLY AS YOU CAN. SAY THIS WORD: TRIANGLE.
18. Repeat MASSACHUSETTS	THE NEXT ONE IS A LITTLE HARDER, BUT TRY TO DO YOUR BEST. SAY: MASSACHUSETTS.
19. Repeat METHODIST EPISCOPAL	NOW REPEAT THIS ONE: METHODIST EPISCOPAL.
20. Write SQUARE (K)	DON'T SAY THIS WORD OUT LOUD (point to item K). JUST WRITE IT ON YOUR PAPER. If the patient prints the word, ask him or her to write it in script or cursive.
21. Read SEVEN (L)	READ THIS WORD OUT LOUD (show item L).
22. Repeat SEVEN	NOW, I WANT YOU TO SAY THIS AFTER ME: SEVEN.
23. Repeat and explain HE SHOUTED THE WARNING	I AM GOING TO SAY SOMETHING THAT I WANT YOU TO SAY AFTER ME. LISTEN CAREFULLY: HE SHOUTED THE WARNING. NOW YOU SAY IT. PLEASE EXPLAIN WHAT THAT SENTENCE MEANS. Sometimes the examiner will have to ask for additional explanations by asking the kind of situation to which the sentence refers. The patient must indicate that danger is impending.
24. Write HE SHOUTED THE WARNING	NOW, WRITE THAT SENTENCE ON THE PAPER. The sentence can be repeated if necessary.
25. Compute 85 − 27 = (M)	HERE IS AN ARITHMETIC PROBLEM. COPY IT ON THE PAPER AND TRY TO SOLVE IT (show item M).
26. Compute 17 x 3 =	NOW DO THIS ONE IN YOUR HEAD. HOW MUCH IS 17 x 3?
27. Name KEY (N)	WHAT IS THIS? (Show item N).
28. Demonstrate use of KEY	SHOW ME HOW TO USE THIS IF YOU HAD ONE IN YOUR HAND (show item N).

Table 7.1 *(continued)*

29.	Draw KEY (N)	NOW, PLEASE DRAW A PICTURE THAT LOOKS LIKE THIS ONE. TRY TO MAKE YOUR KEY LOOK ENOUGH LIKE THE ONE IN THE PICTURE SO THAT SOMEONE WOULD KNOW IT WAS THE SAME KEY AS IN THE DRAWING (point to item N).
30.	Read (O)	WOULD YOU READ THIS? (show item O).
31.	Place LEFT HAND TO RIGHT EAR	PLEASE DO WHAT IT SAID.
32.	Place LEFT HAND TO LEFT ELBOW	NOW, I WANT YOU TO PUT YOUR LEFT HAND ON YOUR LEFT ELBOW. The patient should realize that this is not possible.

Note: From Boll, T. J. (1981). The Halstead-Reitan neuropsychological battery. In S. B. Filskov & T. J. Boll (Eds.), *Handbook of clinical neuropsychology*. New York: Wiley-Interscience. Copyright © 1981. Reprinted by permission of John Wiley & Sons, Inc.

by Salter, Jutai, Foley, Hellings, and Teasell (2006) in their review of aphasia screening instruments following stroke, although there are a variety of aphasia screening tests to choose from, there is little freely available published material on these instruments. For example, the Frenchay Aphasia Screening Test (FAST) was developed as a tool for noncognitive specialists to identify language impairments with a 3–10-minute assessment (Enderby & Crow, 1996). The Sheffield Screening Test for Acquired Language Disorders (SST; Al-Khawaja, Wade, & Collins, 1996) was subsequently developed, and is highly correlated with the FAST as an instrument that does not require special equipment or stimulus cards. The Mississippi Aphasia Screening Test (MAST) was designed to be used as a repeatable screening measure for individuals with severely impaired language skills; it only requires 5–10 minutes to administer (Nakase-Thompson et al., 2005). Although the clinical utility of these instruments is limited, they have the potential to provide a fast and somewhat reliable assessment of aphasic symptoms.

The Token Test

The Token Test examines the ability to comprehend and follow single and multistep verbal commands. It is very easy to administer and score.

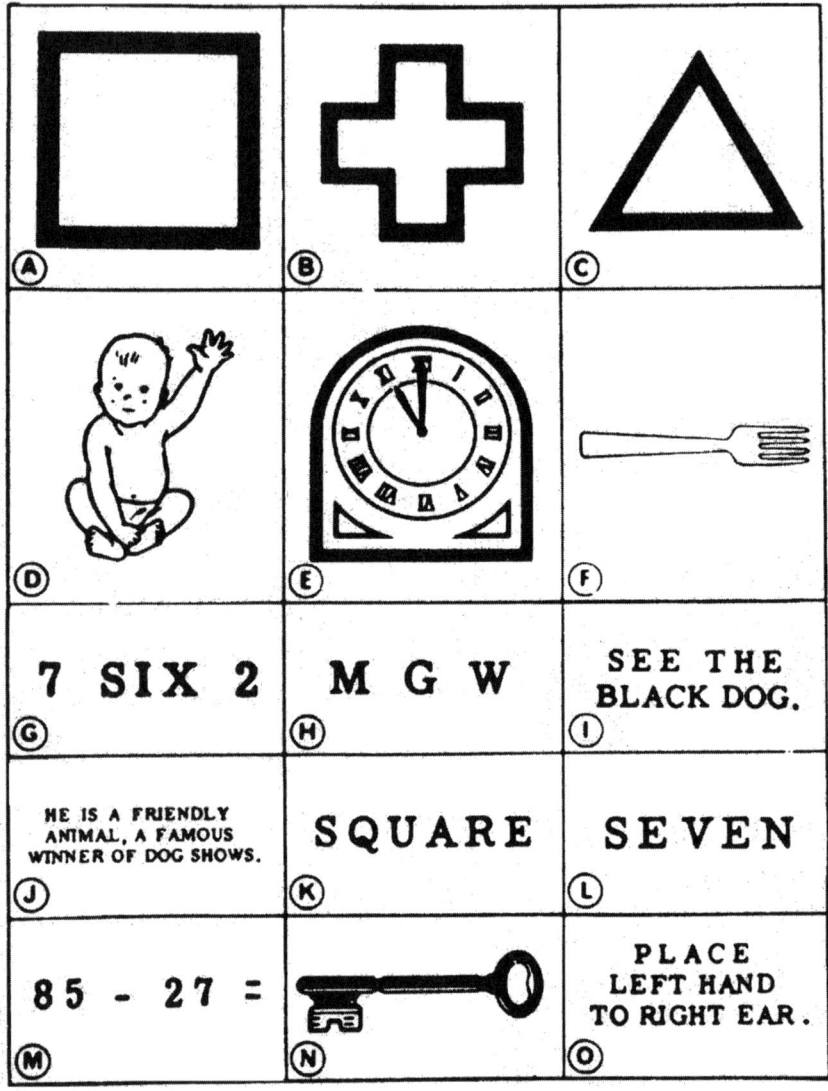

Figure 7.1. Stimulus figures for testing cerebral functions.
Note: From Boll, T. J. (1981). The Halstead-Reitan neuropsychological battery. In S. B. Filskov & T. J. Boll (Eds.), *Handbook of clinical neuropsychology* (p. 593). New York: Wiley-Interscience. Copyright © 1981. This material is reproduced with the permission of John Wiley & Sons, Inc.

The test is composed of 20 items that come in two shapes—circles and rectangles; two sizes—large and small; and five colors—red, yellow, blue, green, and white. Patients are required to understand the token names, as well as the verbs and prepositions, in the instructions (i.e., "pick up the small red circle"). In the original version, there are a total of 62 instructions divided into 5 sections, with increasing complexity of instruction from one section to the next.

Although the Token Test is relatively easy to administer, it is important that the examiner maintains a consistent rate of instruction delivery, regardless of the patient's performance. Any item failed on the first section of the test should be repeated. Only the performance on the second administration is counted toward the overall score, as initial errors may be a result of nonaphasic variables, such as inconsistent concentration or lack of effort. Each correct response earns 1 point, with the highest possible score being 62.

The Token Test has been shown to be effectively administered to a nonaphasic patient who has completed fourth grade with few, if any, errors (Boller & Vignolo, 1966; DeRenzi & Vignolo, 1962). Almost all patients with brain damage can respond to the simplest level of instructions on the test (Lezak, Howieson, & Loring, 2004). It can be used to identify affected linguistic processes that are a part of aphasic disorders, even when the patient can communicate effectively. The test can also identify aphasia in brain-damaged individuals whose other cognitive impairments may interfere with recognizing a language disorder.

There are multiple shorter versions of the Token Test. With an optimal cutoff score, Boller and Vignolo (1966) were able to correctly identify 100% of normal individuals, 90% of patients without language disorders but with right-hemisphere lesions, and 65% of aphasic patients. Cross-validation on another sample resulted in significant shrinkage (Hartje, Kerschensteiner, Poeck, & Argass, 1973). Strauss, Sherman, and Spreen (2006) offer a somewhat different version of the Token Test. Using their scoring method, the test becomes sensitive to even minor impairments of receptive language. The last section (Part 5) of the original Token Test, consisting of items involving relational concepts, was found to correctly identify only one fewer patient as aphasic than did the entire 62-item test. Benton (1994) has a similar 22-item version as part of the Multilingual Aphasia Examination. The Meyers Short Battery (Volbrecht et al., 2000) includes a version of the Token

Test adapted by Spreen and Benton (1977) that uses a slightly altered version in which the rectangles are replaced with squares and includes a total of 39 commands. This version of the Token Test has been found to have a 96% correct classification rate of mild traumatic brain injury from non-traumatic brain injury participants (Meyers & Rohling, 2004).

Tasks that are similar to the Token Test are found on subtests of more comprehensive language evaluations, such as the Clinical Evaluation of Language Fundamentals. The Computerized Revised Token Test is adapted from McNeil and Prescott's (1978) Revised Token Test.

NAMING

Confrontational naming is the ability to use the correct word during speech. Dysnomia, the inability to name objects correctly, occurs when lesions occur in the left temporal lobe for right-hand-dominant individuals (Hamberger, Goodman, Perrine, & Tamny, 2001). Dysnomia is associated with numerous etiologies with various levels of impairment. Because there is a high incidence of naming difficulties in language disorders, as well as in other neuropathological conditions, many language assessments contain a confrontational naming task.

Boston Naming Test

The Boston Naming Test (Kaplan, Goodglass, & Weintraub, 1983, 2001) is a very popular, well-standardized 60-item test designed to offer a detailed examination of naming abilities. There are 60 black-and-white drawings with both high- and low-frequency vocabulary words. The drawings are presented one at a time, and if the client does not produce the word within 15 seconds, prompting cues, including a phonetic cue and providing the beginning sound, are given. The most recent edition includes a recognition component of the test, as well as a 15-item short version. Detailed test administration procedures and scoring instructions are included in the test manual. There are numerous studies providing good normative data for elderly persons, adults, and children (Cruice & Worrall, 2000; Heaton, Avitable, Grant, & Matthews, 1999; Ivnik, Malec, & Smith, 1996; Mitrushina, Boone, Razani, & D'Elia, 1999; Tombaugh & Hubley, 1997).

VERBAL FLUENCY

It is not uncommon for individuals to demonstrate decreased speed and amount of verbal production following injury to the brain. Although impaired fluency alone does not necessarily reveal the presence of aphasia, it is an indicator that can be assessed quickly and effectively. A fluency problem may occur in speech, writing, or reading. More often than not, all three activities will be affected. There are a number of techniques for checking verbal fluency in the course of a screening for possible brain dysfunction.

Controlled Word Association Test

The production of spoken words beginning with a designated letter has been extensively examined by Benton and his colleagues. The associative value of each letter of the alphabet, with the exceptions of X and Z, was determined in a normative study using control subjects who were not brain injured (Borowski, Benton, & Spreen, 1967). Although there are many techniques asking for the generation of words, the Controlled Word Association Test (COWA) is commonly used. The COWA consists of three word-naming trials using the letters, F, A, and S, respectively. The examiner asks the client to say as many words as he can think of that begin with the given letter of the alphabet, excluding proper nouns, numbers, and the same word with a different suffix, including "ing," "er," or "est." The score is the sum of all correct words pronounced in the three 1-minute trials, adjusted for age, sex, and education. The adjusted scores are then converted to percentiles. For example, individuals with less than 12 years of education receive a minimum of five word-increased adjustment regardless of age or gender. Similarly, adults 60 years or older receive an adjusted increase of at least three words, regardless of the amount of education they have earned. However, older adults (>60) with less than 9 years of education receive an adjustment of approximately 13 words. The adjusted scores are then converted to percentiles. After these adjustments, a raw score above 30 words is considered average, with a standard deviation of approximately 7 words.

Categorical Fluency

Another assessment of speech production and amount is categorical fluency. In this test, individuals are asked to produce as many different words as they can think of that fall within a certain category for 60 seconds. Common categories include animals, fruits and vegetables, and items found in a grocery market. Research has found that categorical fluency is less difficult than letter fluency in healthy participants (Mitrushina, Boone, Razani, & D'Elia, 1999) and depressed patients (Hart, Kwentus, Taylor, & Hamer, 1988). However, the impairment of semantic knowledge about categories leads Alzheimer's and Parkinson's patients to have more difficulty with category fluency, compared with letter fluency (Fama et al., 1998). This distinction explains, in part, the rationale for categorical fluency being incorporated in screening instruments used to assess dementia, such as the Mattis Dementia Rating Scale–2 (Jurica, Leitten, & Mattis, 2001).

WRITING FLUENCY

There are many components of written language that can indicate fluency-related impairments. A specific screening test examining writing fluency is the Primary Mental Abilities Test (Thurstone, 1938; Thurstone & Thurstone, 1962). This test examines the patient's ability to write as many words as possible within a specified time. The task requires the patient to write as many words as possible beginning with the letter S within a 5-minute time limit. Next, the client is asked to write as many four-letter words beginning with "C" as he can in 4 minutes. The average individual can produce 65 words within the 9-minute total writing period (Lezak, Howieson, & Loring, 2004). Milner (1967) found that the performance of individuals with left-frontal lobectomies was significantly impaired on this test, when compared with patients whose surgery was confined to the right hemisphere. Cohen and Stanczak (2000) found that the test had limited discrimination ability.

READING FLUENCY

The Stroop Test

The Stroop Test (Stroop, 1935) can be used as a measure of verbal fluency as well as a general test of cognitive efficiency. Materials for the Stroop include three white cards, each of which contains 10 rows of 5 items. Randomized color names—blue, green, and red—are in black print on the first card (A). Card two (B) is identical to the first, except that each color name is printed in some color other than the one it names. Card C displays colored dots in the same array of three colors. There are three trials, each consisting of a different task. On the first trial, the patient reads Card A. During trial two, the patient is asked to read the names of the colors on card B; for trial three, she is asked to name the color of the ink on card C. Throughout the three trials, the patient is instructed to read or name colors as fast as possible. Stroop tasks are also commonly found on the Internet.

Golden (1978) developed another version of the Stroop Test, demonstrated to be useful in identifying brain damage. This version consists of three 8½-by-11-inch pages. Each of 100 items on the first page is one of the following words: red, green, or blue. These words are repeated on the page in a random order. The second page also consists of 100 items, but each item is the sequence XXX. On this page, each XXX is printed in red, green, or blue ink. The third page consists of the words from page 1 printed in the colors used on page 2; however, a word and the color in which it is printed do not match. Therefore, "red" can be printed in either blue or green ink, "green" in red or blue ink, and "blue" in red or green ink.

The instructions for page 1 require that the patient read down each column as quickly as possible, pronouncing the words. For page 2, the basic instructions remain the same, except that the patient is told to name the color of the XXX. Finally, on the third page, the patient is instructed to name the color of the ink, rather than the word itself. Forty-five seconds are allotted for each page. The score is the number of items correctly finished within the time limit on each page. These scores are then converted into standardized T-scores using tables in the test manual.

This version of the Stroop was found to differentiate reliably among normal, psychiatric, and brain-damaged patients. On page 2, normal patients were able to complete 70–90 items, psychiatric patients completed 60–80 items, and brain-damaged individuals were able to complete less than 60, on average (Golden, 1976). Golden (1979) notes that this version of the Stroop can be used to localize lesions: good performance on pages 1 and 2 in conjunction with poor performance on page 3 is characteristic of frontal lobe dysfunction, especially on the left side. Patients with damage to the right hemisphere tend to perform normally on page 1, but poorly on pages 2 and 3. Left-hemisphere damage that is not located in the frontal regions tends to lead to poor performance on all pages of the test.

The Stroop has also been found to be useful in the identification of dyslexia. Equivalent scores on pages 2 and 3 are never seen in literate adults (Golden, 1979). Thus, if the page-3 score is within 10% of the page-2 score, there is a high possibility of dyslexia, as this implies that the normal interference problem (words interfering with color naming) has not occurred, and that there is a lack of word-reading responses.

ACADEMIC SKILLS

It has been noted that few neuropsychological batteries or screening tests contain measures of academic skills, such as reading, writing, or arithmetic (Lezak, Howieson, & Loring, 2004). Examining these areas is important, as impairment can contribute to functional difficulty in occupation and other areas of life. There are a variety of easily and quickly administered academic-skills assessment devices available, such as the *Wide Range Achievement Test-IV* (WRAT-4; Wilkinson & Robertson, 2006).

The *WRAT-4* is a norm-referenced test that measures basic academic skills. It is standardized on 3,000 individuals ranging from 5–94 years. It can be administered in less than 25 minutes to children, and in 30–45 minutes for older participants. It is comprised of four subtests: word reading, sentence comprehension, spelling, and math computation. A Reading Composite score can be derived that is reported to be a highly reliable and comprehensive measure of reading achievement. It also has alternate forms that can be used interchangeably.

The *Gates-MacGinitie Reading Tests, Fourth Edition* (GMRT; MacGinitie, MacGinitie, Maria, & Dreyer, 2000) are paper-and-pencil multiple-choice tests in four primary levels, as well as three grade and high school levels. The *GMRT* measures different aspects of reading, including vocabulary and comprehension.

Other, more extensive academic measures include the *Wechsler Individual Achievement Test, Second Edition* (WIAT-II, Wechsler, 2002) and the *Woodcock-Johnson III Tests of Achievement* (WJ-III; Mather & Woodcock, 2001). Both of these tests have multiple subtests examining areas of academic functioning, including reading, mathematics, spelling, and writing. Whereas these tests differ in length and content of subtests, both are intended to be used to assess academic competency. In doing so, they allow for the evaluation of language-based skills such as grammar, spelling, pronunciation, fluency, and comprehension.

CONCLUSIONS

Intact language abilities are important for communication. Although assessment of some language-based difficulties is easily completed through observation, the scope of language abilities is wide. This allows for a wide range of possible language impairments. Although general screening instruments can evaluate for possible aphasia, clinicians must be aware of the numerous possible language difficulties and that no screening instruments will adequately assess all aspects. If language deficits are observed during a screening procedure, a thorough evaluation by a specialist is recommended, as it is likely to be associated with an underlying neurological disorder.

8 Screening Tests for Memory Functions

A disruption of memory functioning is a common complaint that accompanies a wide variety of clinical conditions and, as such, has many potential causes. Memory is not a unitary construct. Therefore, a screening of memory functioning should cover the span of immediate memory, the addition of new information to recent memory, the extent of recent memory, and the capacity of the individual for new learning (Lezak, Howieson, & Loring, 2004). Ideally, these different memory functions would be systematically reviewed through the major input and output modalities with both recall and retrieval techniques. However, in those cases in which memory problems do not seem to be primary in nature, thoroughness can be sacrificed for a number of practical considerations such as time, patient cooperation, and fatigue.

With most adults, the *WAIS-IV* (*Wechsler Adult Intelligence Scale–Fourth Edition*; Wechsler, 2008) is a generally good starting point. It directly enables the examiner to assess the span of immediate memory, as well as the extent of remote memory (via the Information subtest) stored in verbal form. The longer Arithmetic and Comprehension subtest questions also offer the clinician indirect information on the duration and stability of the immediate verbal memory trace. The mental status examination (MSE; described in detail in chapter 5) can augment information gathered from the patient with a delayed verbal memory task, requiring the patient to recall three spoken items after 5 minutes of intervening material, as well as with questions to assess the retention of ongoing experience at the minimal level necessary for independent living. The addition of an immediate memory and retention task, using simple designs, and a test of learning ability will offer a more complete review of the major dimensions and modalities of memory.

When performance on these tasks is not significantly depressed relative to the patient's best performance on other tasks, and particularly when performance on tests of remote memory is not significantly better than the handling of learning tasks, the clinician can make the assumption that memory and learning are reasonably intact. Pronounced deficits on the general review of memory may suggest the need for a more in-depth memory assessment, which involves the systematic comparison between functions, modalities, and the length, type, and complexity of content. This can be done by the clinician doing the screening if she has had the appropriate training and time is available, or it may point to the need for the patient to be referred out for a comprehensive evaluation of cognitive functions.

A relatively poor performance only on tests of immediate memory and learning may indicate that the patient is severely depressed, and may suggest the need for such a differential determination. Impaired immediate memory and learning are also common early symptoms of a variety of neurological conditions that can ultimately result in general cognitive deterioration. As the still relatively intact patient with neurological dysfunction experiences his failing abilities, he may also be appropriately depressed, further compounding the differential diagnostic picture.

VERBAL MEMORY AND LEARNING PROBLEMS

There are many techniques that can be used to screen for verbal memory and learning problems. The almost unlimited possibilities for combining different kinds of verbal stimuli with input and output modalities and presentation formats have resulted in the development of numerous verbal memory tests. Many of them were developed in response to specific clinical problems or research questions. Our discussion of specific assessment tools will be limited to those few tests and standardized batteries that have been consistently demonstrated to be useful to the clinician.

The clinician's choice of memory screening tests depends on clinical judgment, rather than on scientific demonstration that any given test is most suitable for answering a specific question. Even with the many tests available, the examiner may occasionally find that none will suit the needs of a specific patient, and may be required to devise his own individual memory test for screening purposes. The experienced clinician also may wish to use portions of existing batteries to address specific types of memory difficulty.

Digit Span

The Digit Span subtest of the *WAIS-IV* (Wechsler, 2008) is the most widely used test of verbal immediate memory. The test has two general sections, both consisting of seven pairs of random sequences of numbers. In the Digits Forward segment, the examiner reads aloud number sequences that are from three to nine digits long, and the patient must repeat each segment exactly as it is heard. The Digits Backward portion of the subtest operates in much the same fashion, the major difference being that the patient must say the digits read by the examiner in reverse order. Each section of Digit Span discontinues when the patient fails to repeat both number sequences of a pair of equal length.

This test produces three scores: Digits Forward, Digits Backward, and total Digit Span. The Forward and Backward scores are the number of digits in the longest correctly repeated sequence for each section. The total Digit Span score is the sum of the scores of the two sections. All but a few elderly individuals are able to recall at least four digits forward and three backward, but less than 1% achieve the maximum nine forward and eight backward. The average adult will be able to recall six digits forward and five backward.

In addition to immediate auditory–verbal memory, Digit Span involves auditory attention. The Digits Backward segment of the test measures not only immediate memory, but also the capacity of the patient to juggle information mentally. The ability to reverse sequences effectively requires both memory and the reversing operation to operate simultaneously, a kind of mental "double tracking" (Lezak, Howieson, & Loring, 2004). The fact that Digits Forward and Digits Backward do not involve identical operations is apparent in the score discrepancy of three or more points between the Forward and Backward segments that tends to occur in brain-damaged patients with concentration problems. This is not a common response pattern of brain-damaged individuals who do not have difficulties with concentration, and is rarely seen in non-brain-damaged persons (Costa, 1975).

The immediate memory assessed by the Digit Span test tends to be more vulnerable to left-hemisphere dysfunction than to either right-sided or diffuse injury. This vulnerability is reflected in factorial studies of brain-damaged and elderly individuals in which, contrary to the results of factor analytic studies of normal groups, a verbal factor contributes significantly to the test performance, whereas the prominence of a memory factor is reduced, but not nullified.

Rey Auditory-Verbal Learning Test

The Rey Auditory-Verbal Learning Test (RAVLT) is a brief, easily administered, paper-and-pencil task that assesses immediate memory span, new learning, susceptibility to interference, and recognition memory. The original version was developed by Rey (1964), and was later adapted for use with English-speaking individuals. It has been used in multiple clinical settings and populations, as well as being a frequent research instrument. There are multiple versions in terms of words used and in terms of procedures. Additionally, there are versions available in different languages, including Hebrew (Pollack, Kahan-Vax, & Hoofien, 2008). This versatility makes it attractive for use in a general clinical setting. The clinician who wishes to add this instrument to his/her armamentarium should be careful that the version used is the same as the one for which the norms and cutoff scores have been derived. The RAVLT may also be useful in discriminating between the memory impairment associated with neurologic disease versus psychiatric disorder (Schoenberg et al., 2006). It possesses reasonable test–retest reliability that increases its utility in conducting serial evaluations to determine possible changes (Delaney, Prevey, Cramer, & Mattson, 1992).

The test starts as a test of immediate word memory span. For the first trial (of six), the examiner reads a list of 15 words at the rate of one per second. Before beginning the list, the patient is told that he will be read a word list, and then be asked to repeat as many as he can remember, in any order, when the examiner stops. The examiner writes down the words recalled by the patient. The patient's pattern of recall can be tracked, in order to examine whether the patient is able to cluster words according to category. If the patient asks the examiner whether a word has already been said, the patient should be told. After the patient is finished recalling words, the examiner gives a second set of instructions and then rereads the list. The second set of instructions informs the patient that the same list will be read again, and that when it is completed, the patient is to say back as many words as can be remembered. The patient is also asked to repeat the words said the first time and told that the order is not important.

The list is reread for trials III, IV, and V, using the second-trial instructions each time. Praise may be given as words are recalled, and the patient may be told the number of words recalled, especially if the patient is able to use the information for reassurance or as a challenge. On the completion of the last trial, the second word list is read, with instructions similar to those for the first word list. Following the reading of the second-list trial, the patient is asked to recall as many words from the first list as he can (trial VI). Should either the first- or second-list presentations be spoiled by interruptions, improper administration, confusion, or premature response on the patient's part, the third word list is available. Following a 20-minute delay, which should be filled with other activities, the patient is then asked to recall as many words from the first list (list A) as he can. Once the delayed-recall task is complete, the examiner then asks the patient to identify from printed lists (recognition) as many words as he can from both lists A and B.

The score for each trial is the number of words correctly recalled. A total score, the sum of trials one through five, can also be calculated. Words that are repeated can be noted, as can words that were not on the list (errors or confabulations). Normative data are available for ages 16–89 (Schmidt, 1996).

Hopkins Verbal Learning Test–Revised

The Hopkins Verbal Learning Test–Revised is a 12-word list-learning task. The 12 words are organized into 4 semantic categories. There are 3 learning trials, followed by an unwarned 20-minute delay recall and a recognition task. Brandt and Benedict (2001) provide normative data that was subsequently also published in the test manual. There are six alternate forms, with good reliability on the free recall portion. This allows for serial evaluations.

Selective Reminding Test

The Selective Reminding Test (SRT) was first described as a specific procedure to measure verbal learning and memory during a multiple-trial learning task by Buschke (1973; Buschke & Fuld, 1974). Although there is no commercial source for this test, it is highly effective in assessing memory functioning (Spreen, Sherman, & Strauss, 2006). The stimulus material consists of a list of words, index cards containing the first two to three letters of each word on the list, and index cards containing the multiple-choice recognition items. The procedure requires that the examiner read the patient a list of words, and that the patient recall as many of these words as possible. Each subsequent learning trial involves the selective presentation of only those items not recalled on the immediately preceding trial. The SRT distinguishes between short- and long-term components of memory by measuring recall of items that were not presented on any given trial. The learning rate of patients can also be assessed. Several different versions of the test have been developed (e.g., Hannay, 1986; Hannay & Levin, 1985), including a children's version. The three constructs of Short-Term Recall (STR), Long-Term Recall (LTR), and Consistent Long-Term Recall (CLTR) have shown reasonable validity (Delaney, Prevey, Cramer, & Mattson, 1992). Modifications of the original procedure include learning until two consecutive correct trials are achieved (Chiaravalloti, Balzano, Moore, & Deluca, 2009), and using 8, rather than the original 12, trials (Smith, Goode, La Marche, & Boll, 1995).

The total test administration time for the test is about 25–30 minutes for adults and 10 minutes for children. Scoring the test is somewhat more complex than average, and may take the new user a bit of practice to feel comfortable. If a word is recalled on two consecutive trials, it is assumed to have entered long-term storage (LTS) on the first trial. Once a word enters LTS, it is thought to be in permanent storage and is recorded as LTS on all subsequent trials, regardless of the patient's subsequent recall. When a word in LTS is recalled, it is scored as a long-term retrieval (LTR). When a word in LTS is consistently recalled on all subsequent trials, it also is scored as consistent LTR (CLTR) or list learning on the first of the uninterrupted successful recall trials. Inconsistent LTR refers to recall of a word in LTS followed by subsequent failure to recall the word. It is scored as random LTR (RLTR). STR refers to recall of a word that has not entered LTS. The total recall (Sum Recall) on each trial is the sum of STR and LTR. The number of reminders given by the examiner before the next recall attempt is equal to 12 (Sum Recall of the previous trial). Record by number the order of the patient's recall on each trial (see Exhibit 8.1). Intrusions of words not on the list also are recorded for each trial. (As noted, the scoring is complex, but practice does make it easier.) Full scoring instructions, word lists, and other information are available in the publications referred to earlier.

VISUAL MEMORY FUNCTIONING

Memory can also be examined through nonverbal or visual means. Given the reliance of language, measuring nonverbal memory can be challenging. As such, many of the visual memory tasks that are used are a part of larger assessment batteries. A brief sample of visual-based memory tasks are listed in the text that follows.

To minimize the possibility of verbal mediation, most visual recall test stimuli consist of designs or nonsense figures. However, unless they are quite complex or unfamiliar, geometric designs do not fully control for verbal mediation. Additionally, it is virtually impossible to design a large series of nonsense figures that do not elicit verbal associations. Often, these tests include a practice response, usually drawing. This, of course, can serve to confound the interpretation of deficient performance, because the patient's failure may arise from a practice deficit, from impaired visual or spatial memory, or from an interaction between these (or other) dysfunctions. Even on recognition tasks that do not call for a practice response, such perceptual defects as visual–spatial inattention may compound assessment of memory difficulties. Therefore, the clinician must pay close attention to the quality of nonverbal memory test performance in order to estimate the relative contributions of memory, perceptual, and practice components to the end result of the patient's performance.

Exhibit 8.1

Buschke Selective Reminding Test Record Form

Name: _____ Date: _____ Patient # _____

Examiner: _____

Trial							1	2	3	4
	5	6	7	8	9	10	11		12	
	CR		MC	30						

throw
flower
film
waver
soft
beet
stream
helmet
smoke
hoed
blank
ton
Reminders
Intrusions

Trial 1

Total Recall	_____	(Number words recalled over 12 trials)
LTR	_____	(Words recalled 2x in a row, assumed to be in LTS from this point on)
		(Underline word with red, counting blanks. Compute over 12 trials)
STR	_____	(Words not underlined. Compute over 12 trials.)
CLTR	_____	(Words not continuously recalled. Mark with highlighter. Sum over 12 trials.)
RLTR	_____	(Words that are underlined by NOT CLTR. Do not count blanks. Sum over 12 trials.)
Reminders	_____	(Compute over 12 trials. Max = 144)
Intrusions	_____	(Sum over 12 trials.)
Cued Recall	_____	(Max = 11)
Multiple Choice	_____	(Max = 12)
30 Minute Recall	_____	(Max = 12)

Brief Visuospatial Memory Test–Revised

This measure quickly assesses visual learning and memory using a three-trials paradigm similar to list-learning tasks. The measure is designed for the presentation of 6 figures on 1 page for 10 seconds. There is no time limit for the recall. Following a 25-minute delay, the patient is asked to reproduce the design again. Benedict (1997) designed this task to measure immediate recall, learning rate, delayed recall, and recognition abilities. This test includes six different forms to allow for serial testing. Subtle practice effects have been found (Benedict & Zgaljardic, 1998).

Rey-Osterrieth Complex Figure Test

As mentioned in chapter 6, the Rey-Osterrieth Complex Figure Test requires the patient to copy a complex figure, prior to reproducing the figure 3 minutes and 30 minutes later. As well as assessing visual–spatial construction abilities, the measure is also used to assess visual memory. It is recommended that other tests require drawing or examination of visual designs not be administered during the delay component.

Tactile Memory—The Tactual Performance Test

This test uses the Sequin-Goddard Formboard, which, although originally a visuopractic task, was converted by Halstead (1947) into a tactile memory test by administering it to blindfolded subjects and adding a drawing recall segment to the test. Reitan incorporated this version of the test into his testing battery. Three trials are given in Halstead's administration. Each of the first two trials is done with each hand used singly, with the preferred hand being used first. The third trial uses both hands. The score for each trial is the time to completion (getting all the blocks into the proper holes while blindfolded) in seconds. On completion of the formboard trials, and after the board and the blocks have been removed from the patient's view, the blindfold is removed from the patient. The patient is then given a blank sheet of paper and a pencil and instructed to draw from memory as much of the board as is remembered, and to indicate the different shapes and their locations relative to one another on the board. Two scores are obtained from the drawing. The memory score is a simple count of the number of shapes reproduced with reasonable accuracy (e.g., a star without the correct number of points still receives credit as long as the basic star shape is preserved). The location score is the total number of blocks placed in proper position relative to the other shapes and the board.

MEMORY TEST BATTERIES

To provide a thorough coverage of the varieties of memory disorders, several batteries of memory tests have been developed. These test batteries attempt to examine various aspects of memory with consideration of contemporary theories on memory functioning. The normative data is based on the administration of the entire battery. However, it is not uncommon for some subtests, rather than an entire battery, to be administered for screening purposes. Only qualified professionals trained to conduct the entire battery of tests should do so.

Wechsler Memory Scale–IV

Of all the memory test batteries that have been developed, the various iterations of the *Wechsler Memory Scale* (currently the *WMS-IV*; Wechsler, 2009) have possessed the most systematic normative data and the largest amount of clinical research. The *WMS-IV* is the most recent version in a venerable tradition of memory-assessment instruments. As such, the research base is more limited than for the earlier versions, but that is likely to be a temporary condition. The *WMS-IV* contains six subtests. One subtest, Verbal Paired Associates, may substitute the learning task of the California Verbal Learning Test-II.

The first section of the *WMS-IV* consists of a brief MSE. Three of the subtests (Logical Memory, Verbal Paired Associates, and Visual Reproduction) are similar to subtests found in the earlier versions of the *WMS*. Logical Memory tests immediate recall of verbal ideas from two paragraphs that are read to the patient. This form of test assesses immediate free recall following auditory presentation. Each paragraph read to the patient contains memory units or "ideas," and the patient is given one point for each "idea" that is recalled, with the total score being the number of ideas recalled for each paragraph.

Visual Reproduction is an immediate visual-memory drawing task. Various designs are shown to the patient for 10 seconds, after which she draws the design from memory as completely as possible. Such tests are particularly sensitive to right-hemisphere damage. McFie (1960) found a significant number of impaired design reproductions associated with right-hemisphere lesions, regardless of the specific site of the lesion. This deficit was not found, however, in patients with left-hemisphere damage.

The Verbal Paired Associates subtest taps verbal retention. This task consists of word pairs that are read to the subject, following which the first word in each pair is told to the subject and she is asked to recall the second word in each pair. Generally, patients with left-hemisphere injury tend to do less well on this type of task than do patients with right-hemisphere lesions.

The newer subtests include Symbol Span, in which the subject is shown a linear series of symbols for 5 seconds. Then, the subject is shown a larger set of symbols and asked to point to the target symbols in the same order as the linear array. The next subtest, Spatial Addition, involves showing the subject a grid with blue, red, or both blue and red dots, and then showing a second grid. On a grid without dots, the subject is asked to place a blue card where blue dots were located, or a white card if a blue dot was in that spot in the grid for both previous grids. Finally, for Design Memory, the subject is shown between four and eight designs on a grid and then handed cards with designs. The subject is asked to point to the designs and the spots on the grid in which they were seen. There are both immediate recall and delayed recall procedures.

Wide Range Assessment of Memory and Learning–Second Edition

The *Wide Range Assessment of Memory and Learning–Second Edition* (WRAML-2) was revised from the original version in 1990. Sheslow and Adams (2003) included index scores of Attention and Concentration, as well as eliminated a Learning Index, in the second edition. The WRAML-2 has a core battery of tests that includes six subtests: two attention/concentration, two verbal, and two visual subtests. These six tests compose a General Memory Index score, as well as Attention/Concentration Index, Verbal Memory Index, and Visual Memory Index. There is a variety of optional subtests that can be administered, as well. Further, a screening battery of four Core Battery subtests can be administered to evaluate verbal and visual memory.

Rivermead Behavioural Memory Test

The *Rivermead Behavioural Memory Test* (*RMBT-III*; Wilson, Cockburn, & Baddeley, 1985) differs from most other published tests of memory in its direct attempt to sample memory functioning that is characteristic of everyday life, rather than the traditional doctor's-office learning-and-memory tasks typified by the other memory tests. The RBMT is notable for its attempt to provide a somewhat more meaningful and ecologically valid assessment of memory over the course of time.

Mattis Dementia Rating Scale

The Mattis Dementia Rating Scale (Mattis, 1976, 1988) was designed to provide a quick index of cognitive function in subjects with known or suspected dementia. It includes items similar to those employed by neurologists in bedside MSEs. The items are arranged hierarchically, so that adequate performance on an initial item allows the examiner to discontinue testing within a section, and assume credit can be given to the patient for adequate performance on the subsequent tasks. The subtests include measures of attention (digit span), initiation and perseveration (performing alternating movements), construction (copying designs), conceptualization (similarities), and verbal and nonverbal short-term memory (sentence recalled and design recognition). There is now a revised version with updated norms (Jurica, Leitten, & Mattis, 2001). Additionally, there is an alternate form (Schmidt, Mattis, Adams, & Nestor, 2005), for which reasonable validity has been reported (Schmidt, Lieto, Kiryankova, & Salvucci, 2006). Administration time is about 10–15 minutes for normal elderly individuals. Spreen, Sherman, and Strauss (2006) note that the test can clearly differentiate brain-impaired patients from normal elderly individuals. The instructions and scoring procedures are not as precise as would be desired; however, the test was designed as a screening device and, as such, works well.

CONCLUSIONS

Evaluating memory is a particularly relevant component of cognitive screening, as memory problems are often the complaint of the patient. Assessing various aspects of memory, including, but not limited to, immediate recall, learning abilities, and LTR in both visual and verbal capacities, allows the clinician to assist in diagnosis and treatment planning. Although there are a variety of memory tasks, we have presented a sample of the more commonly used tests.

9 Screening Tests for Higher Cognitive Functions

In addition to assessing specific neurocognitive content areas, such as memory or visuoperceptual functioning, screening for cognitive impairment may take the route of assessing a higher-order skill, or assessing across multiple skill areas, by sampling relevant content areas. An example of the former would be the Wisconsin Card Sorting Test (WCST; Heaton, 1981), which requires intact skills in multiple areas for successful performance. Impaired performance on the WCST may be the result of dysfunction in any number of constituent skills. The Folstein Mini-Mental State Examination (MMSE; Folstein, Folstein, & McHugh, 1975; discussed earlier) would be an example of the latter situation, in which only a few items related to orientation, memory, arithmetic calculation, language comprehension, and construction are administered in order to determine whether impairment exists.

This type of broad screening instrument exhibits a magnification of the generalizability challenge present in all psychological assessments. The best (most accurate) neuropsychological test is life. However, we use tests as samples of relevant behaviors in order to draw conclusions and make predictions about behaviors in the open environment. In a comprehensive neuropsychological evaluation, we administer multiple items but minimize the number of items to economize the amount of time required. There is a trade-off between completeness and efficiency.

In broad-range screening instruments, there may only be one item for each cognitive content area. Although specificity may be adequate, this may be at the expense of sensitivity.

The evaluation of higher cognitive skill typically occurs through the use of executive functioning measures. *Executive functioning* is a term used to describe problem solving, planning, organization, inhibition, and a variety of other behaviors thought to be controlled by frontal and subcortical processes. There are many symptoms of limited executive functioning, including concrete thinking. Concrete thinking prevents the ability to think abstractly about problems and limits problem-solving skills. Further, cognitive rigidity and/or inflexibility may prevent a person from adapting to changes in his or her environment, preventing the successful ability to alter his or her approaches to various problems.

Conceptual concreteness and cognitive rigidity are sometimes treated as different aspects of the same dysfunction. When they occur together, they tend to be mutually reinforcing in their effects (Lezak, Howieson, & Loring, 2004). Although both are associated with extensive or diffuse injury, significant conceptual inflexibility can be present without the inability to form and apply abstract concepts, particularly when there is damage to the frontal lobes (Zangwill, 1966). Additionally, concreteness does not imply impairment of specific reasoning abilities. Thinking may be concrete even if the patient is able to perform such specific reasoning tasks as making practical judgments. Conversely, when the patient has specific reasoning disabilities, thinking is likely to be concrete (Lezak, Howieson, & Loring, 2004).

Executive-functioning impairment occurs in many populations in a variety of ways. For example, individuals with attention deficit disorder may have limitations in their ability to inhibit behavior. In comparison, individuals with traumatic brain injury may have difficulty with problem solving. Interpretation of results of these tests should always be done in the context of a complete history.

Most tests for assessing higher cognitive processes are limited in understanding various executive-functioning capabilities. Typically, these measures examine one or few components of higher cognitive processes. Arguably, the most thorough evaluation of executive functioning is the Delis-Kaplan Executive Functions System or D-KEFS (Delis, Kaplan, & Kramer, 2001), which is composed of nine tests of higher order function. Although the original intent of the D-KEFS is to provide an assessment of executive function in the context of a comprehensive neuropsychological evaluation, some of its subtests might be used in isolation as screening tests. Some of the tests (Color Word Interference, Verbal Fluency, Trail Making, Proverbs, Design Fluency, Tower) are modifications of other, more familiar, tests. The benefit of using the D-KEFS versions here includes procedures to decompose the errors and access to the normative base. Some of the tests are relatively novel. The Sorting test involves two-dimensional cardboard stimuli with various attributes along which they might be sorted or grouped (e.g., size, color, type of object). The test is open-ended in time, and the subject is asked to sort the stimuli as many different ways as they can determine. Because of the open-ended time, this might not be time-efficient regarding the meaning of a nonsense word. With each succeeding piece of information, the subject is asked to guess the identity of the nonsense word. For the Twenty Questions subtest, the subject is shown an array of objects depicted on a page. The subject is instructed to ask yes or no questions to eliminate as many nontarget objects as possible, in order to identify the target object. The score is the number of questions required and the abstraction level of each question.

TESTS OF CONCEPT FORMATION

Tests of concept formation differ from most other executive-functioning tests, in that they focus on the quality or process of thinking more than on the content of the response. A number of these tests have no correct answer, per se. Scoring is done through qualitative judgments of the extent to which the response was abstract or concrete, complex or simple. Tests with right and wrong answers might belong in the category of tests of abstract conceptualization, to the extent that they yield information about how the patient thinks.

Patients with moderate to severe brain damage or with a diffuse injury tend to do poorly on tests of abstract thinking, regardless of the mode of presentation and response. However, individuals with mild, modality-specific, or subtle dysfunction may not engage in concrete thinking generally, but do so only on those tasks that directly involve the use of an impaired modality, are highly complex, or impact on emotionally laden content.

Proverbs Test

Several tests ask the patient to interpret proverbs as a way of evaluating the quality of thinking. Tests such as the Wechsler scales, the Stanford-Binet scales, and a standard mental status examination (MSE) include proverb-interpretation items. The Proverbs Test (Gorham, 1956) is a formal standardized test of proverb interpretation. The standardization of the task reduces variations in administration and scoring biases, and provides normative data that account for the difficulty level of the individual proverbs. There are 3 forms, each with 12 proverbs that are purported to have equal difficulty. The subject is asked to write an interpretation of the proverb. A sufficiently abstract interpretation earns two points, whereas a concrete interpretation earns one point. If the gist of the proverb is missed entirely, the subject is given no points. The mean scores for each form of the test do not differ significantly.

There is also a second multiple-choice version of the test that contains 40 items, each of which has four alternative explanations for the proverb. Only one of the alternatives is appropriately abstract; the remaining choices are either concrete interpretations or common misinterpretations.

Scores on the Proverbs Test tend to vary with education and social class (Gorham, 1956). A study by Benton (1968) using the multiple-choice version of the test with frontal-lobe-diseased patients found these patients perform very poorly on this task, achieving a mean score of 11.4. On the multiple-choice form of the test, both schizophrenic and brain-damaged patients performed significantly more poorly than did normal control subjects; however, the two patient groups could not be differentiated from one another (Fogel, 1965).

Abstract Words Test

Tests that require abstract comparisons between two or more words can provide a sensitive measure of concrete thinking. The clinician must remember, however, that such tests are very dependent on the integrity of the patient's language skills, intelligence, and educational background.

The Abstract Words Test (Tow, 1955) calls for comparisons between two words. The patient must tell how the words differ from one another. For example, *poverty* and *misery* and *abundance* and *excess* are word pairs that the patient is asked to differentiate. There is no formal scoring for this test. Rather, the clinician must make a qualitative judgment of the appropriateness of the patient's response.

A similar form of test is the Similarities subtest of the Wechsler scales. In this test, however, the patient is required to tell how the words are the same. Scoring is done using a system detailed in the *Wechsler Adult Intelligence Scale (WAIS-IV)* manual (Wechsler, 2008). Patients tend to find this test somewhat more difficult than the Abstract Words Test noted earlier, as it is usually easier to tell how things differ than how they are the same.

Sorting Tests

Another approach to evaluating abstract reasoning and concept formation is through sorting tests. In sorting tests, the patient is required to determine how various objects "go together." Often, the patient is asked to sort collections of items, including blocks, cards, or tokens. The directions to these tests are limited, which provides the patient the opportunity to demonstrate abstract reasoning skills and concept abilities on an unstructured test. Interpretation of the patient's skills includes both objective performance and subjective evaluation and observation, such as whether the patient is able to sort according to a rule.

Although sorting tests demonstrate how the patient thinks and handles certain types of abstraction problems, they have not been shown to be useful in differentiating brain-damaged from psychiatric patients (Goldstein & Scheerer, 1941). On scored tests, few significant differences have been found between the mean scores of normal controls and brain-damaged patients (Newcombe, 1969). Thus, a sorting test by itself will not prove to be an effective screening test, but it can be quite useful when administered in conjunction with other tests.

Color Sorting Test

This simple, nonverbal sorting test by Goldstein and Scheerer (1941) consists of 61 little skeins of wool, each of which is a different combination of hue, shade, and brightness. There are about 10 skeins in each of the major colors—green, red, blue, and yellow, plus shades of gray, brown, purple, and other combined hues. The test requires the patient to (a) sort the sample; (b) match two or three different skeins, two of which are similar in hue and two in brightness; (c) explain the underlying principle of sameness in grouping six skeins of the same hue but different shades, and six skeins of different hue but the same brightness; and (d) select all of the skeins of the same hue, such as "blue" or "red," giving his reasoning for the selection. The clinician judges the patient's level and his ease of abstract thinking from both observations and the patient's accompanying explanations.

Color Form Sorting Test

Sorting tests that include a requirement to shift concepts offer more information than simple sorting tests, such as the Color Sorting Test. Observation can help to clarify whether the patient's primary deficit is in sorting or in the shifting of cognitive set.

The Color Form Sorting Test (Weigl, 1941) is made up of 12 tokens or blocks colored blue, red, yellow, or green on one flat surface, and all white on the opposite surface. The tokens or blocks come in three shapes (circle, square, and triangle) and are laid before the patient with the colored side up. The patient is first asked to sort the test material in any manner that is thought to be appropriate. When the patient completes the first sorting, she is then told to group them again, but in a different way. Upon completion of each sort, the examiner asks the patient to explain the reasoning behind the sorting that has just been completed. If the patient has difficulty in a second attempt at sorting, the examiner can offer clues, such as turning all blocks so that the white side is up if the patient's first sort was by color. If the patient performed the first sort by shape, the examiner can show the patient a single grouping formed by color and ask the patient if she can see why the blocks belong together. Impaired mental functioning may be reflected in difficulty shifting sorting principles.

A modification of this test increases the number of possible sorts to five, using thickness, size, and "suit" (a club, heart, or diamond printed at the center of the block), in addition to the four standard colors and three common shapes (DeRenzi, Faglioni, Savoiardo, & Vignolo, 1966). The first part of the test proceeds in the same manner as the original version of the test, except for a 3-minute time limit. When the patient is unable to make an acceptable sort within the 3-minute limit, the examiner makes each of the sorts not used by the patient and allows the patient 1 minute to determine the sorting principle used. Spontaneous patient sorts earn three score points each; correct classification of the examiner's sort receives one point. Scores can range from 0 to 15. Forty control subjects were found to attain a mean score of 9.49. Patients with aphasia performed quite poorly on this modified version of the test, although patients with other types of brain injury did not appear to perform much differently from the normal group. This suggests (as do other studies of sorting tests) that left-hemisphere dysfunction may result in relatively poorer performance on such tasks.

Object Sorting Test

The Object Sorting Test (Goldstein & Scheerer, 1941) is based on the same principles, and generally follows the same administration procedures as are used on the block and token sorting tests, with the exception that the materials used consist of 30 common objects, such as a knife, screwdriver, fork, and so forth. The objects can be grouped according to such principles as use, situation in which they can normally be found, color, material of which the objects are made, and so on. Variations on the basic sorting task require that the patient find objects compatible with the one preselected by the examiner, to figure out a principle underlying a set of objects grouped by the examiner, to sort objects according to a category named by the examiner, or to pick out one object of an examiner-selected set of objects that does not belong to the set. In some instances, the patient may be asked for a verbal explanation. Because the responses are open-ended, the Object Sorting Test allows greater opportunity to evaluate the patient's conceptual style by providing information regarding the qualitative aspects of the patient's responses.

Vygotsky Concept Formation Test

The modified Vygotsky Concept Formation Test (Wang, 1984) is yet another sorting test. There are 22 small wooden blocks with different shapes, colors, widths, and heights. The patient is asked to sort the blocks into four groups. Feedback regarding whether the sort was correct is given following each sort. Following a completed correct sort, the patient is then asked to identify the principle by which the sort was made. As in the other tests discussed in this section, qualitative aspects of the patient's performance are important for interpretation.

Wisconsin Card Sorting Test

The WCST was devised to study "abstract behavior" and ability to "shift set" (Berg, 1948; Grant & Berg, 1948). The patient is given a pack of 64 cards on which are printed one to four symbols—star, cross, circle, or triangle—in green, red, yellow, or blue. The patient is asked to match the cards to one of four stimulus cards—one red triangle, two green stars, three yellow crosses, and four blue circles—according to a principle that the patient must deduce from the pattern of the examiner's responses to the patient's placement of the cards. The responses from the examiner are first organized along matches to color. After 10 consecutive correct placements, the examiner changes the principle being used for placement from color to form, and then after 10 further consecutive responses, the examiner changes the correct principle to number. The test is discontinued after six correct categories are achieved, or when the patient has made six runs of ten correct placements, or when all 128 cards are used (Heaton, 1981). There is also a computerized version of this task.

The WCST is sensitive to a wide variety of cognitive deficits. Frontal-lobe dysfunction may result in difficulty forming abstract concepts. As well, perseveration may be seen in patients with frontal-lobe dysfunction, either as the result of localized lesions or as the result of a history of alcohol abuse. Parsons (1975) describes another type of common error, known as "difficulty in maintaining...set." Here, the patient loses track of the current principle before reaching the criteria of 10 consecutive sorts to principle.

Of note is that Chelune and Baer (1986) present norms for children, and Spreen, Sherman, and Strauss (2006) offer normative data for individuals aged 60–94. In general, by roughly 10 years of age, a child's performance is comparable with that of a young adult (Walsh, Groisser, & Pennington, 1988). Performance on the WCST appears not to significantly decline until after the age of 80 (Spreen, Sherman, & Strauss, 2006). A 64-item version of the WCST has been developed that has been tested on older individuals with comparable results (York Haaland, Vranes, Goodwin, & Garry, 1987).

Category Test

The Category Test (Halstead, 1947) is another test of abstraction ability. Stimulus figures, which vary in shape, size, number, intensity, color, and location and are grouped by abstract principles, are projected on a screen. The patient must figure out the principle underlying stimulus subsets and respond by pressing the appropriate key on a simple keyboard. Correct responses are indicated by a bell, which sounds automatically, and incorrect responses result in a harsh buzz. The test consists of 208 items divided into seven subsets. The patient is told only that each subtest contains a single principle. Correct responses to the first few items are generally a matter of luck. However, the patient should quickly learn the pattern of bells and buzzes, and modify responses by developing and testing new hypotheses until the correct principle underlying the subtest is discerned. The patient is told at the end of each subset that a new subject is about to begin, in which the underlying principle may be the same or may be different from the last subset. Lezak, Howieson, and Loring (2004) note that the test has excellent discrimination ability between brain-damaged and neurologically intact groups. A cutoff score of 50 errors is generally considered to be the point at which cognitive dysfunction is suggested.

The Category Test requires a significant amount of time to administer. Sherrill (1985, 1987) has reviewed three abbreviated versions of the Category Test, and has reported that a 120-item version correlated highly (0.98) with the longer version, with a small standard error of estimate. However, the utility of evaluating memory using the Category test is reduced by consideration of other tests devoted to memory.

ORGANIZATIONAL AND PLANNING ABILITIES

Practical and conceptual organization, ordering, and planning involve an appreciation of the categories and relationships of that which is organized, regardless of whether the organization is to be done using objects, situations, concepts, activities, or any combination of these. Cognitive flexibility, or the ability to recognize alternative solutions, is required, as well as the ability to conceptualize change from present circumstances. There are a limited number of tests that fully capture these abilities. However, observation regarding the patient's behavioral approach to many standard screening tests can be used to assist in understanding how the patient handles these conceptual functions. For instance, the layout of the Bender Visual-Motor Gestalt designs on the page indicates the patient's awareness of space usage and spatial relations. Responses to story-telling tasks can reflect the handling of sequential verbal ideas. The patient's approach toward highly structured tasks allows the examiner to observe the tactical approach to various tests.

Common types of planning tasks are maze tasks. Maze tasks, such as the Porteus Maze test (Porteus, 1965), require patients to plan their navigation of unfamiliar mazes, with or without time constraints. These types of tasks require planning, visual–spatial skills, and visoumotor abilities. These tasks are predictive of brain disorders, particularly for frontal-lobe injuries. Maze tasks are also administered on the computer as well, as discussed in a later chapter.

Information regarding planning can also be obtained through the clinical interview, in which questions concerning the patient's daily activities and future plans can yield indications as to organizational and planning abilities. Lezak, Howieson, and Loring (2004) note that some patients, particularly those with nondominant hemisphere lesions, may give lucid and appropriate responses to questions involving organization and planning of impersonal situations or events, but may show poor judgment in making unrealistic, confused, and often illogical or nonexistent plans for themselves. Such individuals may lack the judgment to recognize that they need to be able to make plans in order to remain independent.

There are other measures that are typically used to assess for various aspects of executive functioning, including the Stroop Color Word Test, Trail Making Test, and the Controlled Oral Word Association Test. These tests have very good normative data, have been extensively studied in a variety of populations, and are discussed in other areas of this book.

Estimation of Premorbid Functioning

Although evaluation of premorbid functioning is important across various cognitive domains, understanding pre-existing higher cognitive skills is particularly important when assessing patients. Ideally, all patients would be tested at some point before the onset of their brain dysfunction, preferably just prior to the event. If this were to occur, then it would be a simple matter for the clinician to compare premorbid and postmorbid test data to determine the extent of dysfunction. Unfortunately, we do not live in such a world, and most patients seen by clinicians do not have premorbid testing data available. Matarazzo (1990) notes that there are several clinical, medicolegal, and research situations in which knowledge of premorbid IQ is important. Several clinicians and investigators have relied on the Vocabulary and Information subtest scores of the Wechsler scales as the best indicators of premorbid functioning. Although the Vocabulary subtest is among the most resistant to change of the Wechsler subtests, and performance on the test can significantly decline as a result of a large range of clinical conditions (Spreen, Sherman, & Strauss, 2006). The Vocabulary subtest is thus likely to underestimate premorbid intelligence (Crawford, 1992; Lezak, Howieson, & Loring, 2004). Although the Information subtest score can reflect a person's general fund of knowledge, it can be misleading in patients with poor educational background and opportunities. It has been argued that a reading test for irregularly spelled words is a better indicator of premorbid ability, as it would assess the reading level achieved before the brain dysfunction (Nelson, 1982). The National Adult Reading Test (NART) was developed in Britain to test this hypothesis. The NART is composed of 50 irregular words such as naive and debt, and has good internal and test–retest reliability. Crawford (1992) notes that the NART does provide a better estimate of WAIS-R IQ than Vocabulary subtest scores. NART performance does deteriorate in patients with severe cerebral dysfunction (Stebbins, Wilson, Gilley, Bernard, & Fox, 1990). Although NART performance can indeed, therefore, be affected by cognitive impairment, it may provide a lower limit to a premorbid IQ score estimate (Stebbins, Wilson, Gilley, Bernard, & Fox, 1990). An adaptation for use with a North American population version of the NART was developed by Blair and Spreen (1989), and is available in the public domain for use (Spreen, Sherman, & Strauss, 2006).

Using demographic measures to estimate premorbid IQ functioning has also offered promising results, with occupation, education, and race being the most powerful predictors (Spreen, Sherman, & Strauss, 2006). Numerous investigators have developed regression equations to calculate premorbid IQ (e.g., Barona, Reynolds, & Chastain, 1984; Reynolds & Gutkin, 1979). Table 9.1 shows the Barona Index formulae

Table 9.1

BARONA IQ ESTIMATE EQUATIONS

Estimated verbal IQ = 54.23 + 0.49 (age) + 1.92 (sex) + 4.24 (race) + 5.25 (education) + 1.89 (occupation) + 1.24 (urban–rural residence)
Standard error of the estimate = 11.79; $R = 0.62$

Estimated performance IQ = 61.58 + 0.31 (age) + 1.09 (sex) + 4.95 (race) + 3.75 (education) + 1.54 (occupation) + 0.82 (region)
Standard error of the estimate = 13.23; $R = 0.49$

Estimated full-scale IQ = 54.96 + 0.47 (age) + 1.76 (sex) + 4.71 (race) + 5.02 (education) + 1.89 (occupation) + 0.59 (region)
Standard error of the estimate = 12.14; $R = 0.60$

Variable weights (to be substituted in the preceding equations)

Sex: 1 = female; 2 = male   *Race:* 1 = other; 2 = black; 3 = white

Occupation: 1 = unskilled labor
2 = semiskilled labor
3 = not in labor force
4 = skilled labor
5 = managerial/office/clerical/sales
6 = professional/technical

Region (U.S.): 1 = South; 2 = North Central; 3 = Western; 4 = Northeast

Residence: 1 = rural (< 2,500); 2 = urban (> 2,500)

Age: 1 = 16–17; 2 = 18–19; 3 = 20–24; 4 = 25–34; 5 = 35–44; 6 = 45–54; 7 = 55–64; 8 = 65–69; 9 = 70–74

Education (years): 1 = 0–7; 2 = 8; 3 = 9–11; 4 = 12; 5 = 13–15; 6 = 16+

Note: From Barona, A., Reynolds, C. R., & Chastain, R. (1984). A demographically based index of premorbid intelligence for the WAIS-R. *Journal of Consulting and Clinical Psychology, 52,* 885–887. Adapted by permission.

and variable weights. It is important to remember that the resulting indices are estimates of premorbid ability rather than exact indicators. An estimated premorbid full-scale IQ above 120 or less than 69 may result in significant overestimation or underestimation (Sweet, Moberg, & Tovian, 1990).

CONCLUSIONS

The evaluation of higher cognitive functioning has long been an interest of neuropsychologists. Numerous tests have been developed to assess different areas of higher cognitive functioning. Impairment can occur in abstract reasoning, problem solving, planning, organization, or other facets of executive functioning in most clinical populations. As a result, functional impairment in daily living is not uncommon. Quickly assessing these different areas is impossible. The clinician must use her clinical judgment to determine which areas of executive functioning are a concern in order to adequately screen for impairment. If there is any uncertainty, or any difference is noted between performance on a screening test and clinical information that is provided, a thorough evaluation of executive functioning is recommended.

10 Neuropsychological Screening

SCREENING VERSUS SINGLE TESTS, VERSUS COMPREHENSIVE ASSESSMENTS

Comprehensive neuropsychological assessments, such as the Halstead-Reitan (Reitan & Wolfson, 2009), the Luria-Nebraska Batteries (Golden, 2004), and the Boston Process Approach (Milberg, Hebben, & Kaplan, 2009), have been shown for several years to be effective in differentiating brain-damaged from psychiatric and normal patients. As such, it would seem to make sense to administer a complete evaluation to every patient for whom the presence of organic dysfunction is suspected. Careful evaluation of patients seen either in private practice or in outpatient mental health clinics should identify those with brain dysfunction, allowing appropriate treatment, which otherwise might not have been considered, to be instituted. However, not all clinical psychologists or examiners have learned the necessary skills or had the training needed to competently administer and interpret a comprehensive neuropsychological assessment. These skills and knowledge can be readily acquired; however, not all clinicians are willing or able to invest the time and money necessary to develop proficiency in the art of neuropsychological diagnosis and treatment planning. Current guidelines approved by Division 40 of the American Psychological Association (Bornstein, 1991) advise that proficiency in neuropsychology can be attained only after a minimum of 2 years' exclusive and full-time postdoctoral training in neuropsychology under the supervision of a qualified neuropsychologist, and through a graduate degree program with a special emphasis in neuropsychology. Such training is becoming increasingly available throughout the country. There are more graduate training programs in psychology that offer a distinct emphasis in neuropsychology; however, there are still fewer than other clinical training programs. Similarly, there are few such postdoctoral training programs. The competition for the available slots at either the predoctoral or postdoctoral level is keen.

A number of highly competent clinicians feel that they can get the requisite training by attending one or another of the workshops that have proliferated in the past few years to deal with the administration and interpretation of some of the most popular neuropsychological test batteries. However, even those who offer the workshops will admit, and frequently emphasize to those in attendance, that the workshop cannot make one a competent neuropsychologist. What the clinician can gain from these workshops is a knowledge of administration techniques for a given test battery or assessment technique, as well as some very basic knowledge about interpreting the results of the test. The 1-, 2-, or even 5-day workshop does not make the clinician an expert in the plethora of complex subtleties involved in brain–behavior relationships, nor is any substantial information typically given concerning the brain functions and their interrelationships that underlie manifest behaviors. Additionally, as the neuropsychology credentialing boards identify more individuals as competent practitioners, reimbursement for non-credentialed clinicians will become much more difficult to obtain.

A second reason that the private-practice clinician or the clinician working for a mental health center or private hospital may not want to perform comprehensive neuropsychological evaluations is the sheer amount of time involved. In certain circumstances, a comprehensive evaluation can take up to a week, depending on the patient's physical and mental condition. More often, an evaluation will take anywhere from 4 to 8 hours, depending on which assessment technique and supplemental tests are used. The vast majority of practicing psychologists simply do not have that amount of time to devote to a single patient. Psychologists in private practice often depend on treating a comparatively large number of patients in any given day to earn their livelihoods. For them to conduct an occasional neuropsychological evaluation that requires the devotion of a full day does not make economic sense. Practitioners working in mental health settings or in private hospitals with small staffs may be required to see far too many individuals to spend the time required for a neuropsychological evaluation of one patient.

Finally, the cost of the equipment and materials needed to conduct neuropsychological evaluations is frequently prohibitive for only occasional use. A complete Halstead-Reitan Test Battery setup, including all equipment and materials, can cost as much as $2,500 or more at the time of this writing. The Luria-Nebraska Test Battery will cost about $425 in terms of initial costs. Both batteries now have computer-assisted scoring available, which can increase the cost still further, particularly if the clinician buys a computer. Thus, the initial investment can be great, and this cost does not include any additional test equipment, or those materials that are frequently used by neuropsychologists to supplement the information from the more comprehensive batteries. By their very nature, each of the available comprehensive evaluation batteries is, in a sense, nothing more than a comprehensive screening battery that offers the possibility of generating hypotheses about the brain integrity of a patient that may, in turn, require further in-depth investigation with any number of other test instruments.

Thus, to perform neuropsychological evaluations, the clinician really must be willing to devote all of her professional energies to neuropsychology. It is extremely difficult to be a good "part-time" neuropsychologist without either the general clinical practice or the neuropsychological aspect of the practice suffering.

Neuropsychological screening offers a practical alternative to this, because it generally does not require much in the way of special equipment. Administration and interpretation of a screening generally requires far less time than that required for the more complete evaluation. Additionally, the cost in terms of materials and personnel, as well as space, is typically a good deal less. A relatively brief, portable, and easily administered and scored battery of tests is much more practical and cost-effective in those situations in which the primary requirement is to differentiate those individuals who have brain-based pathology from those who do not.

Over the years, a number of investigators have attempted to identify a single test that will differentiate patients with brain damage from non-brain-damaged individuals. In virtually all instances, such attempts have failed, and continue to do so. There is a very simple reason for this: One single test cannot possibly tap all aspects of brain functioning. There are individual tests that are exceptionally good in terms of identifying one form or another of organic dysfunction, such as the Halstead Category Test (described in chapter 9); however, if the patient being assessed does not happen to have a dysfunction in the area being tapped by the test, but does indeed have some form of cognitive impairment, that particular patient may be inappropriately identified as non-brain-damaged. As a very simple and gross example, a patient with language disturbance will likely not be identified as impaired by the Bender Visual-Motor Gestalt; similarly, the patient with a visual–spatial processing disturbance will be classified as normal if just the Speech Perception Test is used as the screening device.

A good neuropsychological screening battery is designed to minimize the time needed for administration, scoring, and interpretation, while maximizing the information gathered by briefly assessing all major cognitive functional areas. These functional areas include lateral dominance; motor functioning; auditory, tactile, and visual sensation; spatial–perceptual organization; language skills; general information; and memory processes. Furthermore, the tests included in such a battery should have as little redundancy as possible, and should be empirically demonstrated to be effective in differentiating brain-damaged from non-brain-damaged individuals. All of the tests included should be brief, easily administered, objectively scored, commonly used in clinical settings, and very portable.

What follows is a description of different screening approaches that have either been reported in professional journals, or discussed at length at professional meetings. All of the batteries that will be described have been demonstrated to be effective in assisting the clinician in differential diagnosis. These screening batteries also conform, in large part, to the criteria described earlier. Most of the screenings discussed consist of tests previously described in this book. Because few of these screening techniques have a formal title, they are discussed and named after the battery developers. In the past few years, there have been several commercially available screening devices introduced. These are also discussed.

ABBREVIATED HALSTEAD-REITAN SCREENING BATTERY, VERSION 1

Golden (1976) has offered a useful abbreviated version of the Halstead-Reitan Neuropsychological Test Battery. Version 1 of the Abbreviated Battery is somewhat longer than Version 2 (described in the following), and requires roughly 1 hour for total administration. It consists of nine tests: (a) Trail Making Test, Parts A and B; (b) the Aphasia Screening Test; (c) the Seashore Rhythm Test; (d) the Speech Sounds Perception Test; (e) the Stroop Color and Word Test; and from the Wechsler Adult Intelligence Scale, the (f) Block Design; (g) Digit Symbol; (h) Similarities; and (i) Object Assembly subscales.

All of the tests in this version of the Abbreviated Battery are administered in the generally accepted manner. Scoring for the Wechsler scale subtests requires use of the age-corrected scale scores. For the Trail Making Test, the total combined time to complete Part A and Part B, in seconds, is the score to be used. On the Stroop Color and Word Test, three scores are generated—the number of items completed on the word, color, and combined word–color pages. Scores on both the Speech Sounds Perception Test and Seashore Rhythm Test are the number of incorrect responses on each test. The Aphasia Screening Test is scored in accordance with the technique of Russell, Neuringer, and Goldstein (1970), which assigns different weights to each item, based on its importance.

All test scores are then compared against what are considered to be cutoff scores for performance within the normal range (see Table 10.1). An impairment index is obtained by calculating the percentage of tests that fall within the normal or impaired range. If the performance falls within the normal range for a specific test, a value of 0 is assigned. If the patient's performance is within the impaired range on a specific test, a value of 1 is assigned. It is then a simple matter to determine whether a majority of the test scores have values in the impaired range. If this is the case, there is a reasonable probability that the patient has organic dysfunction.

Golden (1976) also developed a somewhat more accurate (and complex) method of determining whether a patient's test performance on the Abbreviated Battery, Version 1, falls within the impaired or

Table 10.1

CUTTING SCORES FOR THE TESTS IN THE GOLDEN (1976) ABBREVIATED VERSION OF THE HALSTEAD-REITAN BATTERY

TEST	CUTTING SCORE[a]
Aphasia Screening Test	> 6 points
Speech Sounds Perception Test	> 7 errors
Seashore Rhythm Test	> 5 errors
Trail Making Test–Part A	> 33 seconds
Trail Making Test–Part B	> 87 seconds
Stroop—Word Page	< 87 items
—Color Page	< 59 items
—Color–Word Page	< 32 items
WAIS—Block Design	< 9 scale score
—Similarities	< 9 scale score
—Digit Symbol	< 9 scale score
—Object Assembly	< 9 scale score

[a]Indicating impaired performance.

Note: From Golden, C. J. (1976). The identification of brain damage by an abbreviated form of the Halstead-Reitan Neuropsychological Battery. *Journal of Clinical Psychology, 32*, 821–826. Copyright © 1976, Clinical Psychology Publishing Company. Adapted by permission.

normal range. A single score for each patient's performance is obtained by multiplying the patient's score on each measure by the appropriate, empirically derived coefficient listed in Table 10.2.

All derived products are then summed. If the patient's derived score is greater than 210, impairment is indicated. This technique yielded a hit rate of 71.9%, with an amazingly high correct identification rate of 97% of individuals with left-hemisphere damage in the original research conducted with the Abbreviated Battery, Version 1. Alternatively, the patient's individual test score index (0 or 1) can be multiplied by the general test index listed in Table 10.2, and the resulting products can be summed and compared with the cutoff score of 210.

ABBREVIATED HALSTEAD-REITAN SCREENING BATTERY, VERSION 2

In 1978, an abbreviated version of the Halstead-Reitan Neuropsychological Test Battery was reported in the literature (Erickson, Calsyn, &

Table 10.2

GOLDEN ABBREVIATED BATTERY UNSTANDARDIZED COEFFICIENTS FOR DIFFERENTIATION OF BRAIN-DAMAGED AND NORMAL PERFORMANCE

TEST	COEFFICIENT	INDEX
Seashore Rhythm Test	3.1	41.7
Speech Sounds Perception Test	1.2	5.8
Trail Making Test–Part A	0.3	– 26.8
Trail Making Test–Part B	– 0.2	138.7
Aphasia Screening Test	2.0	– 18.8
WAIS—Similarities	1.1	– 29.2
—Digit Symbol	– 0.5	66.0
—Object Assembly	17.2	48.4
—Block Design	– 4.4	126.1
Stroop—Word	– 0.5	-35.1
—Color	– 1.2	– 13.6
—Color–Word	– 0.1	– 19.7

Note: From Golden, C. J. (1976). The identification of brain damage by an abbreviated form of the Halstead-Reitan Neuropsychological Battery. *Journal of Clinical Psychology, 32,* 821–826. Copyright © 1976, Clinical Psychology Publishing Company. Adapted by permission.

Scheupbach, 1978). Based on that original investigation, McNamara, Wechsler, and Munger (1984) studied the utility of the Abbreviated Battery. The Abbreviated Battery is quite short, and is easily administered in well under 1 hour.

The screening device consists of four basic tests: (a) the Trail Making Test (Parts A and B scored in accord with Russell, Neuringer, & Goldstein, 1970); (b) the Aphasia Screening Test (Russell, 1975, scoring); and the WAIS (c) Block Design and (d) Digit Symbol subtest scale scores. Standard administration and scoring methods are applied to each of the tests. The patient's performance is then compared with the following cutoff scores. An average impairment rating is calculated as follows:

Step 1:

Total Impairment Score = 27.338

+ (1.043 x Trail Making A plus B Russell* rating)

+ (-0.655 x Block Design Scale Score)

+ (1.695 x Russell Aphasia Error Rating)

+ (-0.959 x Digit Symbol Scale Score)

Step 2:

Average Impairment Rating = Total Impairment Score / 12

If the average impairment rating is equal to or greater than 1.55, impairment is suggested. Using this technique, McNamara and associates (1984) were able to correctly classify 84% of the original 90 cases studied into impaired and unimpaired groups. Their work also found a high degree of association between the standard Reitan impairment index calculated from performance on the complete Halstead-Reitan Battery, and the average impairment index obtained from the Abbreviated Battery. The abbreviated battery has been shown to be a better screening tool than the Mini-Mental State Exam (Gonzalez, Dieter, Natale, & Tanner, 2001).

BARRY REHABILITATION INPATIENT SCREENING OF COGNITION

The Barry Rehabilitation Inpatient Screening of Cognition (BRISC; Barry, Clark, Yaguda, Higgins, & Mangel, 1989; Barry, 1991) was developed because of a perceived clinical need to provide reliable information to physicians and rehabilitation treatment teams after a brief consultation with brain-injured patients. Many items were derived from existing instruments, with the intent to consolidate those found to be most useful in treatment planning. The BRISC is divided into eight functional categories, providing the clinician with a broad sample of cognitive functions in approximately 30 minutes. The BRISC can be used as a more general screening device, and failure on a significant number of

---

*Refers to Russell, Neuringer, and Goldstein (1970).

items can reflect the presence of significant brain impairment, which may require further investigation.

The first category, Reading, was designed to separate commonly found problems with visual acuity from visual language processing. A variety of visual–motor, oral–motor, reading, and comprehension problems may be inferred from the patient's performance on the five items comprising this section.

The second category, Design Copy, requires the patient to copy five common geometrical shapes. These shapes also become the basis for immediate and delayed spatial-memory sections when assessing memory. In the Verbal Concepts portion of the BRISC, word pairs are presented, and the patient is asked how each pair is alike and how the words in the pair differ. Additionally, these words are used in the memory section to assess immediate and delayed verbal memory. The fourth category, Orientation, requires the patient to provide typical orientation information. Category V, Mental Imagery, was included, as individuals with brain dysfunction often have difficulty in accurately reporting internal visual representations. In this section, the patient is asked to recite the entire alphabet, and then only those letters with curves in them when printed in capital letters. The sixth category, Mental Control, includes a standard digit-span task (including both forward and backward recitation), as well as a sequential alternation task that is comparable with an oral version of Trail Making, Part B. A measure of Verbal Fluency comprises section 7. The patient is asked to generate lists of groceries and clothing. The final section, Memory, includes four measures of incidental memory for the previously seen geometrical designs and word pairs that were presented earlier.

The initial investigation demonstrated good concurrent validity with accepted measures of cognitive functioning, as well as acceptable reliability. A total score of 135 is possible on the BRISC. Scores below 120 points are considered to be indicative of impaired functioning. It is important for the clinician to remember that the BRISC originally was designed for use with and standardized on an inpatient population. Normative data were gathered from normal adults. Although the concepts that underlie the items can be reasonably expected to apply for non-hospitalized individuals, to date, no data concerning the validity of the BRISC as a screening measure are available, and, thus, the BRISC should be used judiciously.

REPEATABLE BATTERY FOR THE ASSESSMENT OF NEUROPSYCHOLOGICAL STATUS

The Repeatable Battery for the Assessment of Neuropsychological Status (Randolph, Tierney, Mohr, & Chase, 1998), or RBANS, is meant to be a relatively short collection of cognitive tests that could be administered bedside, and used in serial assessment to measure change. There are four alternate forms. The procedures generally tap Language, Memory, Attention, and Visuospatial/Construction skills. The normative data are from individuals aged 20–89. It takes approximately 30 minutes to administer. Schoenberg et al. (2006) provide normative data on the retention rates for older patients, adding to the information already available regarding immediate and delayed recall. The RBANS is becoming increasingly popular, and is likely to see greater empirical evaluation.

NEUROPSYCHOLOGICAL ASSESSMENT BATTERY

The Neuropsychological Assessment Battery (NAB; Stern & White, 2003) is a collection of tests that comprehensively evaluate cognitive function in a set of subtests that can be used as a battery or as stand-alone tests. There are 36 different tests in this collection that are organized into modules centered on 6 skill areas. The normative data is based on individuals between the ages of 18 and 97 years who are stratified by age, education, and gender. Of particular interest to the general clinician is a screening module that takes approximately 1 hour to administer. There is limited information regarding the psychometric properties of the screening module in the manual. Iverson, Williamson, Ropacki, and Reilly (2007) examined the use of the screening module in a mixed neurologic population, and found that a substantial proportion (40%) of their sample performed relatively well on individual tests, indicating the need for greater research with this particular module. Most screening instruments have greater sensitivity than specificity, but this appears not to be the case for the screening module of the NAB.

NEUROBEHAVIORAL COGNITIVE STATUS EXAMINATION

The Neurobehavioral Cognitive Status Examination (NCSE or Cognistat; Kiernan, Mueller, Langston, & van Dyke, 1987; Mueller, Kiernan, &

Langston, 1988; Schwamm, van Dyke, Kiernan, Merrin, & Mueller, 1987; Yazdanfar, 1990) was developed in the mid-1980s as a response to a growing need for a brief assessment of different areas of cognitive functioning. The authors reject the use of a mental status examination (MSE) and other comparable measures that quantify cognitive status with a single score, in favor of a multivariate approach that provides indices for different functional abilities. Instead of evaluating "organicity," per se, the Cognistat was designed to assess neuropsychological functions in a brief manner. The Cognistat addresses five major domains of cognitive functioning—language (comprehension, repetition, and naming), construction, memory, calculation, and reasoning (similarities and judgment)—as well as overall level of consciousness, orientation, and attention. It incorporates a screen, as well as a metric, approach, and allows for the development of a profile of the patient's cognitive functioning in different areas. On the sections with a screening item, if it is passed, the clinician can move to the next section without administering the items that compose the metric portion. Total administration time rarely exceeds 20–30 minutes. The test manual provides some reliability and validity data, as well as some limited normative data.

Section I of the Cognistat is a simple assessment of level of consciousness. If the patient is not fully alert, the test should be discontinued, as interpretation is not meaningful. Section II consists of traditional Orientation questions that the patient must answer. In section III, Attention, the patient is asked to perform a Digit Span (forward) task. The second portion of this section requires the patient to repeat four words just related to him or her. For the four-part Language section of the Cognistat, section IV, a speech sample is obtained in Part 1 from the patient by asking her to describe the action in a picture. Although no score is given for this, it allows for a qualitative assessment of the patient's spontaneous speech. Comprehension (Part 2) is next assessed in this section. The patient is asked to perform one-, two-, and three-step tasks in response to verbal commands. Oral language comprehension and complex motor praxis are both involved in this test. For Part 3, the clinician asks the patient to repeat phrases and sentences after oral presentation. Finally, in Part 4, Naming, the patient is asked to name objects and pictures of objects to visual confrontation. Section V of the Cognistat assesses Construction ability. The screen task involves concentration, visual memory, and construction ability. The patient is presented with a complex visual figure to be drawn after a 10-second presentation. In the metric section, the patient is asked to perform a Block Design task. Section VI investigates memory. The patient is asked to recall the four words presented in an earlier portion of the Cognistat. If needed, the patient is presented with category prompts and, finally, verbally presented recognition lists. The Calculations section (VII) consists of a series of arithmetic computations to be performed mentally after oral presentation. Section VIII, Reasoning, is divided into two parts. Part A, Similarities, is basically the same as the task of the same name on the Wechsler scales. The patient is presented with two words, and required to tell how they are alike. Part B, Judgment, consists of practical judgment questions in the form, "What would you do if...?" All responses are scored according to generally clear criteria presented in the manual. Section scores are summed and combined into a total score. Initial data suggest that it is a highly useful screening device (Costello, Bieliauskas, & Terpenning, 1992; Fields, Starratt, Fishman, Cisewski, & Coffey, 1993).

Because of its brevity and because of the need for screening older patients, the Cognistat is frequently used to screen for dementia. Macaulay, Battista, Lebby, and Mueller (2003) provided age-corrected cutoffs for different subscales of the Cognistat, due to there being a different trajectory of changes for the different cognitive skill areas tapped by the Cognistat. As with other screening instruments, the Cognistat is more accurate in identifying the presence of cognitive impairment than in specifying the etiology. Clinicians should be aware that ethnic minorities may be more likely to miss the screening items on the Naming, Calculation, and Similarities subtests, although performance on the full metric items did not show this difference (Schrimsher, O'Bryant, Parker, & Burke, 2005).

COGNITIVE COMPETENCY TEST

The Cognitive Competency Test (CCT; Wang, 1990; Wang & Ennis, 1986; Wang, Ennis, & Copeland, 1987) was developed to directly assess an individual's cognitive competency in maintaining safe and independent living. Although not a neuropsychological screening device, per se, it is believed that the CCT can be a valuable instrument in a clinician's armamentarium. The CCT incorporates the concept of multidimensionality of cognitive skill, and uses a practical approach by simulating daily living skills. The broad range of skills tapped by the CCT offers the clinician a more representative picture of the cognitive competency of the patient.

The CCT consists of eight subtests, each of which measures a different behavioral–cognitive domain. Subtest 1, Personal Information, asks the patient to write information on a printed form resembling application forms used by banks and public agencies. If the patient is unable to write as a function of a specific motor problem or agraphia, the information can be verbally obtained by the examiner. Card Arrangement, Subtest 2, uses five sets of cards to demonstrate the sequences of baking a pie, preparing a meal, sweeping the floor, and doing laundry. The patient is required to arrange the cards into the proper order to demonstrate his or her knowledge of the sequence of actions needed to perform daily activities. Picture Interpretation, Subtest 3, is designed to require the patient to make use of visually presented information to come to conclusions about interactions of the individuals in the picture. The design of the task is such that the patient must logically deduce events either preceding or following the situation presented in the picture. Memory, Subtest 4, has two sections, immediate and delayed recall. The items to be remembered are practical, with a day-to-day relevance: a grocery list, current prices for bus fare and stamps, and an appointment. Administration simulates real-life situations by providing the opportunity for rehearsal through repeated presentation and delayed recall with interference. Practical Reading Skills, Subtest 5, consists of 10 pictures depicting different settings, such as a railway station, supermarket entrance, telephone directory, and so on. The patient is required to read various simple labels and signs in order to answer a question about the picture. Management of Finances, Subtest 6, is designed to determine the ability to handle the specifics and the mechanics of financial matters, and requires a good deal of accuracy on the part of the patient in executing the details of the test. The task includes sorting mail, deciding bills to be paid, writing a check, and computing a balance. Verbal Reasoning and Judgment, Subtest 7, consists of 10 questions intended to assess the patient's understanding of strategies needed for self-preservation and safety judgment. Route Learning and Spatial Orientation, Subtest 8, consists of maps with different landmarks, and assesses specific types of memory (locations and names of landmarks, as well as memory for routes) and directional orientation and spatial judgment. The task requires the use of visual–

Table 10.3

CCT SCORE CLASSIFICATION

AVERAGE TOTAL SCORE (%)	LEVEL OF COGNITIVE COMPETENCY AND FUNCTIONAL INDEPENDENCE
80 and higher	Total independence
70–79	Mostly independent; occasional assistance may be required
56–69	Partial independence; partial and structured assistance is required
45–55	Varying from partial and structured assistance to stand-by supervision
31–44	Mostly dependent; stand-by supervision required
30 and lower	Total dependence

Note: From Wang, P. L. (1990). Assessment of cognitive competency. In D. E. Tupper & K. D. Cicerone (Eds.), *The neuropsychology of everyday life: Assessment and basic competencies* (pp. 219–231). Boston: Kluwer Academic Publishers. Adapted with kind permission from Springer Science and Business Media.

spatial memory and verbal memory, to a lesser extent, for successful completion.

The scores of the eight subtests are summed to yield an average total score (percentage form) that the authors report to be a robust indicator of the level of cognitive competency. Cutoff scores also are provided for each subtest to assist in the identification of strengths and weaknesses in various cognitive skills. The range of scores and identified competency level is presented in Table 10.3. The initial validation data look good. Comprehensive research is under way to evaluate both the legal and psychological efficacy of the CCT.

MINI-INVENTORY OF RIGHT-BRAIN INJURY

The Mini-Inventory of Right-Brain Injury (MIRBI; Pimental & Kingsbury, 1989) is a 27-item instrument that was designed to be used as a tool for screening cognitive deficits associated with right-hemisphere lesions. As originally conceived, the MIRBI is a relatively

Table 10.4

MIRBI GENERAL ITEM CONTENT

Visual scanning
Finger naming
Stereognosis
Two-point discrimination
Unilateral neglect

Reading comprehension
General reading skills
Spontaneous writing
Dictated writing
Cursive *M*s & *W*s
Serial 7s
11:10 Clock Drawing

Expressing happy voice
Expressing sad voice

Understanding humor
Conversation comprehension
Verbal absurdities
Proverb 1
Proverb 2

rapid screening that highlights areas of deficient processing, and allows clinicians to identify neurocognitive domains in need of further examination using a more comprehensive battery. Test results also can assist in delineating for referral potential areas needing immediate treatment emphasis. The items of the MIRBI assess a variety of right-hemisphere processes, as detailed in Table 10.4.

The MIRBI was originally normed on a patient population with well-documented right- or left-hemisphere cerebral vascular accidents, as well as normal individuals. The test has good initial and cross-validation data (Knight, Pimental, Miller, & McWilliams, 1990; Pimental & Knight, 1991). The MIRBI total score discriminated normal controls from documented lesion groups, with a hit rate of 99.97% in the original validation study and an average hit rate of about 90% in the cross-validation. The MIRBI's short time for administration, portability, and item content selected for sensitivity to right-brain injury combine for an initial screening device of high utility.

THE MIDDLESEX ELDERLY ASSESSMENT OF MENTAL STATE

The Middlesex Elderly Assessment of Mental State (MEAMS; Golding, 1989) has been designed as one of a proliferation of devices to assess cognitive functioning in the elderly. As is the case with the Dementia Rating Scale-2, discussed earlier, the MEAMS was designed to offer the clinician a quick screening of cognitive functioning in older individuals to determine whether additional assessment is required. Specifically, the MEAMS assesses gross impairment of specific cognitive skills in the elderly to differentiate between functional illness and organically based cognitive impairments. The test consists of 12 tasks, and taps a wide range of cognitive domains, including orientation, language, calculation, construction, visual processing, memory, and limited motor functioning. A listing of the specific content areas is presented in Table 10.5. There are two alternate forms that can be used, allowing the clinician to do test–retest to determine gross changes over time. Total administration time is 15–20 minutes, and requires very little training. Reliability data presented in the manual looks promising (interrater reliability = 0.98; parallel form reliability = 0.91). It is important to note that comparatively little normative data are available, and little data concerning the initial standardization sample are presented in the test manual. Clinicians who wish to use this device should do so with caution initially, until a clinical familiarity is achieved.

KAUFMAN SHORT NEUROPSYCHOLOGICAL ASSESSMENT PROCEDURE

The Kaufman Short Neuropsychological Assessment Procedure (K-SNAP; Kaufman & Kaufman, 1994) is designed to be a brief, individually administered, nationally normed measure of mental functioning at three levels of complexity: (a) a lower level of attention and orientation (essentially a mental status section); (b) an intermediate level of simple

Table 10.5

ITEM CONTENT FOR THE MEAMS

1. Orientation—time and place
2. Name Learning (visual–verbal association learning)
3. Naming
4. Comprehension (identify objects from description)
5. Remembering Pictures (recognition memory)
6. Arithmetic (simple calculation)
7. Spatial Construction (copy two geometrical figures)
8. Fragmented Letter Perception
9. Unusual Views (common objects viewed from different angles)
10. Usual Views
11. Verbal Fluency
12. Motor Perseveration (based on verbal contingencies)

Scoring: 1 point for each subtest passed
Maximum score = 12
10–12 points = normal performance
8–9 points = borderline performance
< 8 points = impaired performance

---

memory and perception skills (Number Recall and Gestalt Closure subtests); and (c) a high level of complex intellectual functioning and planning ability (Four-Letter Words subtest). The authors note that the K-SNAP is designed for use with individuals ranging in age from 11 to over 90 years. Administration time is reported to be about 20–30 minutes. The clinician should be aware that the K-SNAP may have limited sensitivity, although it possesses excellent specificity (Donders, 1998).

The K-SNAP comes in a basic American Guidance Systems easel kit that contains the four subtests, a record form containing the items for the Four-Letter Words subtest, as well as space for recording biographical information, raw scores, and derived scores. Detailed instructions and normative data are provided in the test manual.

In the Mental Status Subtest, patients are required to respond to simple questions assessing attention and orientation to the world around them. The Number Recall Subtest is a Digit-Span-type task, with number series ranging from two to nine digits. In the Gestalt Closure Subtest, the individuals are asked to name an object or scene pictured in a partially completed "inkblot" drawing. The final subtest, Four-Letter

Words, requires the patient to determine the "secret word" by studying clues presented and generating decision-making strategies.

The intermediate- and high-level subtest scores are combined to yield a composite score. The two intermediate-level subtests yield a Recall/Closure composite score. An Impairment Index is generated based on the application of a set of diagnostic criteria to the subtest and composite scores of the K-SNAP.

CONCLUSIONS

The clinician is faced with determining which approach is the most appropriate technique when assessing for cognitive impairment. Although screening instruments and single tests can detect some brain-based impairment and can be done quickly, their utility is limited. It is also possible that screening instruments may not be thorough enough to detect subtle limitations. Comprehensive assessments, on the other hand, provide more thorough information, but require more training, cost more, and require more time. The decision is left to the clinician to determine the necessity of a comprehensive evaluation. It is suggested that the use of screening instruments, along with clinical history, medical information, and collateral information, should guide the clinician in making the recommendation for a comprehensive evaluation.

11 Effort and Motivation

The evaluation of effort and motivation has been the focus of an incredible amount of conceptual and empirical scrutiny over the past decade. Developing and evaluating instruments to assess effort on cognitive tests and examine for response bias has become a cottage industry in clinical neuropsychological research. The exact prevalence of malingering is unknown, but it probably varies across different populations and settings. For example, it is likely to be more prevalent in situations in which the outcome of the evaluation has some external motivation for the patient. Such might the case in which disability benefits are at stake, or in which the outcome would allow the patient to gain financial reward or avoid negative consequences. Less-than-optimal effort may be also the result of low internal motivation, such as in severe depression or apathy.

The determination of less-than-optimal effort or frank malingering is a complex clinical decision that requires multiple sources of information, including direct observation, knowledge of the external circumstances surrounding the evaluation, and the use of objective specialized assessment instruments. However, in instances in which the generalist clinician suspects less-than-optimal effort, the use of specifically designed instruments or the calculation of indices from existing test data may help formulate the referral, or even determine whether a referral to a specialist is made. The generalist clinician may use one of these instruments and report the results and suspicions or indicate the rule-out to the specialist clinician.

There are a few important points to remember. First, the term *malingering* is frequently used to describe behavior; however, in the clinical sense, malingering refers to a diagnosis. Malingering occurs when an individual consciously exhibits nonoptimal effort or pathological symptoms in order to achieve some external gain. The diagnoses to rule out malingering include delusional disorder, psychotic disorder, hysterical disorders, severe depression, and factitious disorder. The second major consideration is that the tests that have been developed are frequently called tests of malingering, but in fact, they are tests of effort and motivation. These procedures and indices provide information regarding the likelihood that the clinical data obtained in an evaluation is an accurate reflection of the cognitive or emotional state of the patient.

There are a few clinical aspects in which the suspicion of the clinician should be aroused. The first is the situation in which the evaluation occurs. Does the patient have the potential to gain some external reward based on the results? The patient may start the appointment by stating that she wants the results sent to her attorney, or that she was dissatisfied with the results of a prior evaluation conducted by a different clinician. In the course of taking the history, the clinician should always inquire as to whether any legal proceedings are at stake.

The second aspect is in the behavioral observations of the clinician during the interview and test administration. Did the patient appear to be giving adequate effort? Did the patient exhibit exaggerated effort? Was there an inconsistency in which the patient missed easier items and achieved more difficult items? Was there an inconsistency between the test performance and other sources of information? For example, did the patient come on time to the appointment and successfully find the office, but perform in the severely impaired range corresponding to dementia? Was there an inconsistency, in that performance on tests of attention was severely impaired, but performance on tests of memory that rely heavily on attentional processes was intact? It is important to remember that clinical judgment can be subjective and inaccurate. Clinical judgment is susceptible to interpersonal influence. In general, confidence is negatively correlated with accuracy in clinical judgment.

It is always recommended to complement clinical judgment with objective test data.

SPECIFIC TESTS OF EFFORT

21-Item Wordlist

The 21-Item Wordlist (Iverson, Franzen, & McCracken, 1991, 1994) takes approximately 5 minutes to administer and score. Because of its brevity, this test can be used as a short screening procedure at the beginning of an evaluation. It contains 21 words that are presented orally, following which the patient is instructed to recall freely as many words as possible. The patient is then instructed to identify the target words within a two-alternative forced-choice procedure. True positive rates of identification of experimental malingerers have ranged from 20% to 80%, depending on which cutoff scores were used (Frederick, Sarfaty, Johnston, & Powel, 1994; Gontkovsky & Souheaver, 2000; Iverson & Franzen, 1996; Iverson, Franzen, & McCracken, 1991, 1994). Vickery and colleagues (Vickery, Berry, Inman, Harris, & Orey, 2001) demonstrated that the task has high specificity, but low sensitivity. The 21-Item Wordlist has normative information based on hospitalized substance-abusing patients (Arnett & Franzen, 1997).

Rey Memory for 15 Items Test

Along with his substantial contributions of the Rey Auditory Verbal Learning Test (RAVLT) and the Rey Complex Figure, Rey (1964) presented a method for evaluating potential negative-response bias. This is the granddaddy of all such procedures. However, its accuracy has been surpassed by subsequent developments in the field. Nonetheless, it is a simple procedure with reasonable specificity, although its sensitivity may be limited in more cognitively skilled patients. Similar to the 21-Item Wordlist, the Rey Memory for 15 Items Test (Rey, 1964) can be used at the beginning of the examination as a rapid screen. There are 15 visual items presented in 3 columns and 5 rows. Patients are given the cognitive set that this is a difficulty memory task, and that they will have just 10 seconds to study and memorize the items. The items are arranged in logical sequences (e.g., numbers, letters, and shapes). The most frequently calculated scores are the total number of correct items and the number of correctly reproduced rows.

There are different methods of administration and scoring, and it is important the clinician use the method matching the cutoff scores. The most widely used administration is to request recall immediately after exposure. As mentioned earlier, the test has low sensitivity. Arnett, Hammeke, and Schwartz (1995) provided information related to the performance of both neurologic patients and malingerers.

16-Items Test

The 16-Items Test is a variant on the Rey Memory for 15 Items Test. Paul, Franzen, Fremouw, and Cohen (1992) simplified the stimulus by eliminating the geometric designs and adding one item to the remaining four sets, to make the test simpler and more specific to negative-response bias. Similar to the Rey Memory for 15 Items Test, the 16-Items Test has variable sensitivity, but relatively high specificity to negative-response bias (Iverson & Franzen, 1996). Fisher and Rose (2005) corroborated these results, and found that the 16-Items Test was not necessarily an improvement over the original 15-Items Test.

Symptom Validity Testing

Symptom Validity Testing (SVT) is a relatively simple procedure that can be improvised in situations in which a more formal test may not be available. Originally, it was designed to be used to evaluate subjective reports of impaired sensory function (Pankratz, Fausti, & Peed, 1975), but it has also been extended to evaluate claims of memory impairment (Pankratz, 1983). Patients are given a large number of trials of the task they say they cannot perform. The responses are available in a two-alternative forced-choice response format. Less-than-optimal effort is inferred when performance is below the confidence interval surrounding random responding (50% correct). SVT may be helpful in uncovering gross exaggeration, but not subtle symptom magnification.

Forced-Choice Test of Nonverbal Ability

The Forced-Choice Test of Nonverbal Ability is a modification of the Test of Nonverbal Intelligence. Frederick and Foster (1991) combined the two 50-item forms and modified the test, so that only two choices were available for each item, rather than the four choices in the original version. The result is a 100-item, 2-alternative forced-choice procedure. Less-than-chance performance suggests less-than-optimal effort. The test also provides additional scores, including slope, consistency ratio, and correlation between test performance and item difficulty. These scores appear to be reasonably sensitive and specific to negative-response bias (Frederick, Sarfaty, Johnston, & Powel, 1994). Frederick and Speed (2007) elaborate on interpreting the difference between guessing and malingering.

California Verbal Learning Test

The California Verbal Learning Test (CVLT) includes an evaluation of recognition memory, and can be used to evaluate the possibility of less-than-optimal effort. In fact, the computerized scoring program for the CVLT will provide a score related to the probability of symptom magnification (Curtis et al., 2006).

RAVLT

In general, any memory test that uses a recognition procedure has the potential to offer information regarding effort and motivation. In some instances, the multiple scores derived from a test have been submitted to a discriminant function analysis in order to determine a classification system. King, Gfeller, and Davis (1998) report the result of such an attempt using the RAVLT, with the unfortunate result that only 48% of the cross-validation sample was correctly identified as simulating or actually impaired. Bernard (1990, 1991) reports a discriminant function analysis using both the RAVLT and the Rey Complex Figure, but an attempt by Sherman, Boone, Lu, and Razani (2002) resulted in low specificity (33%), albeit with excellent sensitivity (95%). There have been other methods suggested, such as examining for the suppression of primacy effects in the list learning of malingerers, and comparing free recall to recognition. Neither method was especially effective (Sullivan, Deffenti, & Keane, 2002).

Boone, Lu, and Wen (2005) reported that a combination of recognition indices from the RAVLT could be modestly accurate in identifying less-than-optimal effort. Their method involved subtracting the false positive score from the true positive score, and then adding the number of words recognized from the first third of the test, using a cutoff greater than or equal to 12. This formula resulted in 74% sensitivity and 90% specificity in their sample.

Reliable Digit Span

The reliable digit span is a score derived from the use of the Digit Span subtest of the *Wechsler Adult Intelligence Scale, Third Edition* (*WAIS-III*; Wechsler, 1997). In this procedure, the maximum span forward is summed with the maximum span backward. When that sum is below 7, less-than-optimal effort is inferred. This score has been used in evaluating toxic exposure (Greve et al., 2007) and traumatic brain injury (Axelrod, Fichtenberg, Mills, & Wertheimer, 2006). Babikian, Boone, Lu, and Arnold (2006) suggest that lowering the cutoff to six increases the specificity. The reliable digit span procedure has also been used in patients with chronic pain (Etherton, Bianchini, Greve, & Heinly, 2005).

Test of Memory Malingering

The Test of Memory Malingering (TOMM; Tombaugh, 1996) is a set of 50 simple line drawings of everyday objects. The patient is given a few seconds exposure to each picture, then is asked to choose the original stimulus when contained in a forced choice of pairs of pictures. If the patient makes the wrong choice, he is corrected. Then there is another exposure to each picture and another forced choice, this time with different alternatives. Again, the patient is corrected when the incorrect answer is given. Finally, an unwarned 20-minute-delay recognition task is given. The TOMM has been used in cases of brain injury and chronic pain (Greve, Ord, Curtis, Bianchini, & Brennan, 2008), as well as in post-traumatic stress disorder and mild traumatic brain injury (Greiffenstein, Greve, Bianchini, & Baker, 2008) and in general neuropsychological populations (Ruocco et al., 2008). However, Green (2007) suggested that the TOMM is insensitive to feigned impairment, although the results of this study have been called into question (Greiffenstein et al., 2008).

CONCLUSIONS

In general, the diagnosis of malingering is a complicated endeavor that does not lend itself to a screening process. However, by including measures of less-than-optimal effort or symptom magnification in the screening tests, the clinician can begin to acquire hypotheses regarding the accuracy of the test data obtained. The generalist clinician can then provide those observations and test data to the specialist clinician, who can then use a more comprehensive and detailed assessment of effort and motivation.

12 Computerized Assessments

The use of computer-based tests has gained in popularity in recent years. The last edition of this book did not include a section describing this option. At the present time, the availability of these tests as screening instruments warrants the inclusion of a separate chapter. We will briefly discuss the reasons for the increased use of computer-based tests. We will also describe some traditional paper-and-pencil measures that have computerized options, as well as some tests that were designed specifically for use on a computer. Finally, discussion will include some issues that the clinician needs to be aware of when using computer-based screening assessments, and future possibilities for computer-based examinations.

USE OF COMPUTER TASKS

Interest in computer-based tasks is not a new phenomenon in psychology. Although it was primitive, the original version of the *Wechsler Adult Intelligence Scale* was automated in 1969 (Elwood & Griffin, 1972). Although the present version of the WAIS is no longer computer-based, computerized aspects of a cognitive evaluation are well accepted.

Several reasons exist for the increased use of computer testing. Computerized testing does not require extensive training for the person administering the test. Often, the instructions are provided on the computer for the test taker to read and follow. Without the test administrator being required to learn accurate procedures, there is also less likelihood for invalid results due to administration error. For example, when a computer task is used, the test will be administered the exact same way to every patient. Using computer tests is also beneficial in terms of ease and flexibility regarding where tests can be administered. Typically, the materials for neuropsychological tests are cumbersome, and can be difficult to transport. Therefore, patients are often required to complete testing at the clinician's office. In comparison, computer-based tests can be done in a variety of settings, including at a medical doctor's office, on the sideline or locker room of athletic events, and at bedside. Most computer tests also provide immediate results through a printout of performance. This results in efficiency of interpretation of performance, which leads to faster care and ability to immediately answer referral questions.

The rise of computer-based tests may also be associated with cost-effectiveness. In 1998, Sturges described how practical uses of computers have occurred with the advancement in computer technology for clinical practices. Similarly, although purchasing computer-based tests may initially cost more than materials for traditional paper-and-pencil tests, the ability to reuse the tests ultimately leads to overall lower costs across time. Further, whereas it is important to have somebody supervise the computer tasks that are administered, the level of training for the test administrator can be lower than that of the clinician, advanced student, or psychometrist. Given the recent trend toward environmental friendliness, computer-based tests can also cut down on the amount as well as costs of the excessive paper that is necessary for many paper-and-pencil tasks. Further, computer-based measures have been demonstrated to save 60% in time over traditional measures of cognitive-based evaluation in psychiatric populations (French & Beaumont, 1987).

It can be argued that certain cognitive domains can best be evaluated through the use of computerized testing. For example, computerized continuous-performance tasks most effectively evaluate sustained visual attention. In certain circumstances, computerized tests are the most effective and feasible way to study cognition. For example, the use of computer-based tests in conjunction with functional magnetic resonance imaging (fMRI) leads to a greater understanding of the pathology involved with various disorders. The exclusion of automated visual-based measures would likely result in decreased understanding of neurophysiological pathways responsible for cognitive functioning. Even novel computer tests, such as facial affect recognition tests, have been shown to be effective in helping us to understand neurobiological mechanisms of psychiatric and neurological disorders. Computers are also likely to measure aspects of reaction time more validly than stop watches on traditional measures. Overall, there is increased reliability by reducing scoring error.

COMPUTERIZED VERSIONS OF TRADITIONAL PAPER-AND-PENCIL TESTS

There have been several attempts to convert traditional paper-and-pencil measures into computer-based tests. Many of the measures discussed in previous chapters have been computerized, and some of the results are discussed in the following text. We encourage you to review the other chapters to be reminded of the demands of the original paper-and-pencil tasks if there is uncertainty regarding the purpose of the test. Further, those listed in the following are not intended to be an exhaustive review of all computerized cognitive tests, but rather a sampling of those available for public use with supporting research.

The Category Test from the Halstead-Reitan Neuropsychological Test Battery is the subtest from that battery for which the computerized equivalent has been most extensively studied. It has gone through multiple computerized versions until its current edition, which allows for full automation, with the exception of test instructions (Choca, Laatsch, Garside, & Arnemann, 1987). Attempts have been made to computerize the Trail Making Test from the Halstead-Reitan Neuropsychological Test Battery as well, but it is not commercially available (Salthouse & Fristoe, 1995).

Another traditional neuropsychological measure that has a computerized version is the Wisconsin Card Sorting Test. This is a widely used problem-solving test that has gone through numerous versions. The current version (Heaton, Avitable, Grant, & Matthews, 1999) is extensively used in clinical practice to examine higher-order cognitive skills.

Equivalent measures used to assess intelligence have also been created. The Peabody Picture Vocabulary Test (PPVT) and Raven's Progressive Matrices (RPM) are two commonly used screening measures to examine intelligence. The PPVT has been used as part of evaluations with individuals who suffer from neurological problems (Marchand, D'Arcy, & Connolly, 2002). The computerized RPM has been shown to effectively examine nonverbal reasoning, in comparison with traditional paper-and-pencil measures in healthy volunteers (Gur, Ragland, & Moberg, 2001).

There have been attempts to computerize traditional maze tasks, such as the Porteus Maze Task. Ott et al. (2003, 2008) studied a computerized maze task that relates to driving ability. However, it is not commercially available. Similarly, there are computerized versions of the Token Test that are equivalent to the traditional version, but are not yet available to the public (Eberwien et al., 2007).

Unfortunately, historically, research indicates that computer-based versions of some tests do not provide the same results as the traditional paper-and-pencil tests from which they were developed (Feldstein et al., 1999; French & Beaumont, 1987; Tien et al., 1996). It is possible that the anxiety of some people who are unfamiliar with computers results in a decrease of performance. Conversely, other test takers may become more at ease with the lack of human contact during the evaluation (Luciana, 2003).

COMMERCIALLY AVAILABLE COMPUTERIZED ASSESSMENTS

There have been recent advancements in the development of tests that are designed specifically for computer use. Some of the tests examine one construct, such as attention and/or problem solving; whereas others attempt to examine numerous areas of cognition. Following is a brief representation of the commercially available computerized tests that are familiar to clinicians.

The Conner's Continuous Performance Task (CPT-II) is a measure of sustained visual attention, vigilance, and response inhibition. It requires a patient to press the space bar on a computer every time a letter appears on the computer screen, except for the letter 'X.' It allows for examination of the patient's ability to maintain his or her focus over the course of the 14-minute presentation. The CPT-II is one of the most-used continuous performance tests by professionals, and one of the most frequently used measures of attention by neuropsychologists (Rabin, Barr, & Burton, 2005).

The Iowa Gambling Task (IGT; Bechara, Damasio, Damasio, & Anderson, 1994) requires approximately 20 minutes for completion. The IGT examines decision-making ability through the use of a card game with pretend money. Patients with frontal-lobe damage, particularly in the orbitofrontal regions, have a tendency to persevere on the less advantageous approach toward the task (Fukui, Murai, Fukuyama, Hayashi, & Hanakawa, 2005).

Examination of cognitive skills following concussion has also yielded computer-based tests. For example, the Immediate Postconcussion Assessment and Cognitive Testing (ImPACT; Lovell, Collins, Podell, Powell, & Maroon, 2000) is a computer-based test that measures attention, processing speed, reaction time, and memory. It is currently used by professional sports teams, as well as numerous high school and collegiate teams. In comparison, the CogState (1999) measures reaction time, attention, learning, working memory, adaptive problem solving, and spatial abilities in athletes at risk for concussion. Administration time takes 20 minutes. The HeadMinder (Erlanger, Feldman, & Kutner, 1999) measures reaction time and speed of decision making. All three measures have reasonable test–retest capability, and were designed with the expectation that athletes would be administered the tests on numerous occasions to monitor recovery.

The Cambridge Neuropsychological Test Automated Batteries (CANTAB) were developed to evaluate visual attention, working memory, visual memory, and planning. The CANTAB consists of 12 tasks that can be administered either in succession or separately. Therefore, the time of the task depends on the selection of subtests, which ranges from 3–10 minutes each. The CANTAB has been used in numerous populations, and has demonstrated sensitivity to brain-based disorders (Fowler, Saling, Conway, Semple, & Louis, 2002).

CONCLUSIONS

Although computerized cognitive measures have evolved, most neuropsychological measures remain paper and pencil. As in all areas of science, the progression of technology leads to concerns regarding the use of new tools. As previously mentioned, studies have been inconsistent when examining whether the results from computerized versions of the test are consistent with traditional measures. Therefore, clinicians are hesitant to use measures that may not examine the cognitive domain that is of interest. Further, the initial purchase cost of some tests may be beyond what the clinician would prefer to invest, particularly if there is uncertainty regarding clinical utility. And, although computer tests may, in fact, be less expensive to purchase and administer, the test administration still typically requires somebody to be in the same room as the test taker. It is also not uncommon for computers to malfunction or lose data, as well. Regardless, the use of computerized tests as screening instruments is an easy way to collect some initial information on the patient to determine the need for further referral for a thorough evaluation.

Computerized cognitive tests will continue to play an important role in the advancement of the neurological understanding of disorders (Schatz & Browndyke, 2002). Although novel computer tasks will continue to be created and used to examine various areas of cognitive functioning, new versions of pre-existing tasks will also appear. It is impossible for the clinician to ignore the convenience and potential wealth of cognitive data that can be provided through computer-based tests. In the long term, the advancement of technology likely will lead to commercially available, reasonably inexpensive, virtual-reality tests that will allow for clearer evaluation of functional abilities. Evaluation of a patient's ability to drive, cook, interact with others, and function in a classroom setting and other areas of daily living will likely come from yet-to-be-discovered advancements in technology.

Glossary

abducens nerve—The sixth cranial nerve. Lesions here can result in excessive lacrimation.

ablation—An older scientific technique used to examine brain-based behavior, in which a portion of the brain was destroyed and subsequent behavior was observed.

abscess—A circumscribed infection characterized by a buildup of pus surrounded by a thick wall of cells.

absence seizures—A form of epilepsy, typically found in children, characterized by a brief altered state of consciousness (petit mal seizures).

abulia—Inability to perform voluntary acts or make decisions.

acalculia—See dyscalculia. An acquired reduction in a person's ability to perform arithmetic calculations.

acoustic nerve—The eighth cranial nerve. It has two divisions: the cochlear division, which is partly responsible for the transmission of auditory information to the brain, and the vestibular division, which is responsible for the sense of balance.

acoustic neuroma—A tumor, largely comprised of nerve cells and nerve fibers, that often compromises function of the acoustic division of the eighth cranial nerve.

acromegaly—A chronic disease of the endocrine system resulting in elongation and enlargement of certain bone structures, including the frontal bones and jaw bones. Symptoms include muscular pain, headaches, and sweating.

Addison's disease—A condition resulting from a deficiency in secretion of adrenocortical hormones. Symptoms include anorexia, weight loss, nausea, weakness, and fatigue.

afferent fibers—Neuronal pathways that carry information upward toward the cerebral cortex from peripheral areas of the nervous system.

agnosia—Literally, a condition of not knowing. It is the inability to recognize sensory stimuli. Color agnosia is the inability to recognize colors. Visual agnosia is the inability to recognize objects in the presence of intact visual sensation.

agrammatism—A defect in the syntactical composition of the patient's verbal output. It is characterized by the omission of most relational words, including articles, prepositions, and conjunctions.

agraphia—An acquired condition of impaired or absent writing ability.

akathisia—A condition of extreme motor restlessness. It is accompanied by subjective feelings of anxiety and restlessness.

akinesia—A state of lowered motor activity.

akinetic mutism—A state of wakeful unresponsiveness in which there is no apparent purposeful mental activity. The person appears to be awake, but inactive.

alexia—An acquired inability to read.

Alzheimer's disease—A dementia characterized by progressive mental impairment and by the presence of excessive neurofibrillary tangles and senile plaques.

amnesia—A partial or total impairment of memory functions. *Anterograde amnesia* is a disturbance of memory that follows some etiologic event. It is a disturbance of the transfer of engrams from short-term into long-term memory storage. *Retrograde amnesia* is a disturbance of memory prior to the ecologic event. It is a disturbance of retrieval from long-term storage.

amygdala—A structure of the limbic system, important in memory and in the regulation of emotion.

amyotrophic lateral sclerosis—A condition of muscle weakness and atrophy, with spasticity and hyper-reflexia. It is the result of degeneration of motor neurons of the spinal cord, medulla, and cortex.

aneurysm—A weak wall of a vein or artery that dilates and fills with blood and that may hemorrhage, destroying surrounding neural tissue.

angular gyrus—A region of the cerebral cortex, in the area of the posterior parietal lobe, which is intimately involved in the production of speech.

anisocoria—A condition wherein the pupils dilate unevenly to light.

anomia—Sometimes known as "dysnomia," it is a condition in which the patient has difficulty finding correct words. It is often assessed by a confrontation naming task.

anosmia—Lack of the sense of smell. Although it is sometimes associated with lesions of the olfactory nerve (cranial nerve 1), it is more frequently associated with non-central nervous system dysfunction, such as peripheral disease of the nostrils.

anosognosia—A condition in which the patient is unaware of existing deficits. It occurs despite objective evidence that deficits exist, and is often associated with lesions in the posterior non-dominant hemisphere.

anterior cerebral artery—An artery that originates from the internal carotid artery and principally serves the frontal lobes, corpus callosum, olfactory, and optic tracts.

anterior communicating artery—An artery that originates from the anterior cerebral artery, supplies the caudate nucleus, and helps form the anterior part of the Circle of Willis.

anterograde amnesia—Loss of memory for events that follow cerebral trauma, such as often occurs in head injuries.

anticholinergic drugs—Drugs that interfere with passage of nerve impulses through the parasympathetic nerves.

Anton's syndrome—A form of anosognosia in which the patient is totally blind, but lacks awareness of his blindness.

aphasia—An acquired inability to use certain aspects of language. It can be either an expressive or a receptive language disorder. "Aphasia" is a very broad term that is made more useful by descriptive qualifiers indicating the type of language impairment involved.

aphemia—Nonfluent speech with intact writing skills.

apraxia—Impaired ability to perform previously chained skills in a continuous behavior. *Construction apraxia* is impairment in reproducing patterns; it is assessed by observing drawing and drafting, or by having the patient build three-dimensional objects. *Ideational apraxia* refers to impairment in the idea of the required behavior; it is usually assessed by asking the patient to perform several linked behaviors. *Ideomotor apraxia* refers to the inability to demonstrate motor behaviors that were known in the past; it is assessed by asking the patient to pantomime a task, such as using a can opener or using a pair of scissors.

aprosody—A condition in which the coloring, rhythm, melody, cadence, intonation, or emphasis of speech is impaired. A person with this condition is likely to speak in a monotone, even when relaying affective material.

Aqueduct of Sylvius—A narrow canal, about 3/4 inch long, that connects the third and fourth ventricles.

arachnoid—The middle layer of the meninges. The term means "like a cobweb" and is used because of the delicate nature of the arachnoid.

arachnoid space—The space around the arachnoid layer that is filled with fibrous tissue and acts as a conduit for cerebrospinal fluid.

arteriosclerosis—A disease of the vascular system characterized by cumulative buildup of fatty deposits on the inner walls of veins and arteries.

arteriovenous malformation—Abnormally shaped arteries and veins. It may be only a small tangle of vessels, or a large collection of abnormal vessels occupying a large area.

astereognosis—An acquired inability to recognize an object by the sense of touch. It is assessed by handing an object to a blindfolded patient and asking the patient to identify the object.

astrocytoma—A type of neoplasm that develops from astrocyte cells. These tumors are typically unencapsulated and intracerebral.

ataxia—Loss or failure of muscular coordination. Movement, especially gait, is clumsy and appears to be uncertain. Ataxic patients often sway while walking. Ataxia usually results from an inaccurate sense of position, caused by distorted proprioception in the lower limbs. Difficulty with gait increases greatly when the patient is asked to walk with eyes closed.

athetosis—A movement disorder in which involuntary undulating, or writhing movements, occur. These are called "athetoid movements." They are slower and more sustained than choreiform movements, and are associated with increased muscle tone.

atonia—Complete lack of muscle tone.

atrophy—Shrinkage of (brain) tissue due to loss of neuronal processes.

attention—The capacity of an individual to screen out certain aspects of the environment and to perceive and process other aspects.

auditory nerve—Sometimes called the "vestibular" or "acoustic nerve." It is the eighth cranial nerve and transmits auditory information, and also is involved in the sense of equilibrium. (See also acoustic nerve.)

auditory verbal dysnomia—An aphasic deficit characterized by impairment of ability to understand the symbolic significance of verbal communication through the auditory avenue (loss of auditory–verbal comprehension).

aura—A sensory phenomenon that may precede a seizure.

autoimmune disorders—Impairment of bodily processes by which immunization is effected.

autonomic nervous system—That part of the nervous system concerned with visceral and involuntary functions.

axon—The portion of a neuron that transmits energy from the cell body to the receptors of other neurons.

Babinski response—Extension (instead of flexion) of the toes, on stimulation of the sole of the foot, occurring in persons with lesions of the pyramidal tract.

bacterial infection—Infection by minute, one-celled organisms, which multiply by dividing in one or more directions.

ballismus—An abrupt contraction of the extremities that makes it appear as if the person is flapping or flailing her limbs. It is most commonly seen on one side of the body, in which case it is known as hemiballismus. Ballismus is sometimes associated with hypotonia and chorea.

basal ganglia—The region of the brain located within the diencephalon but below the cerebral hemispheres, including the thalamus, caudate nucleus, and lentiform nucleus.

bifurcation—Division into two branches.

bradykinesis—A motor disorder, frequently seen in Parkinson's disease, which results from rigidity of muscles and which is manifested by slow finger movements and loss of fine motor skills, such as writing.

Broca's area—A portion of the left-frontal lobe intimately involved in the production of speech.

Capgras' syndrome—A rare condition wherein the patient is convinced that persons in his close social environment have been replaced with imposters. It is sometimes seen with non-dominant hemisphere lesions, post-traumatic encephalopathy, cerebrovascular disease, and other neurological diseases, but usually only in the early stages.

carcinoma—A malignant neoplasm (cancer) that tends to infiltrate surrounding tissue and gives rise to metastases.

carotid endarterectomy—A surgical technique for cleaning the vessels carrying blood to the brain.

cataplexy—An abrupt decrease in muscle tone. The person with cataplexy feels as if he has suddenly lost control of his limb(s), and may fall if the lower limbs are involved.

cerebral anoxia—A condition in which the cells of the brain do not receive sufficient oxygen to perform their normal functions.

cerebral palsy—A general term for a large number of congenital neurological disorders. The symptoms include movement disorders, weakness, spasticity, and ataxia. Some degree of mental retardation may also be present. The cause is usually some event that occurs during or shortly after the birth process.

cerebrovascular accident—An ischemic disorder that is produced by a disruption of blood flow in the brain due to an occlusion of a portion of the vascular system from a thrombus or embolus, or from a hemorrhage.

chorea—A sudden involuntary movement that serves no apparent purpose. These movements are known as choreiform and are brief in duration. They are asymmetric and can often be masked by the afflicted individual unless the examiner is extremely watchful. They are associated with decreased muscle tone.

clonic movements—Spasmodic alteration of contraction and relaxation, such as is seen in certain forms of epilepsy.

coma—A condition of profound stupor or unconsciousness.

computerized axial tomography—A neurodiagnostic technique in which X-rays measuring densities of sections of the brain are integrated by a computer.

concussion—A form of closed-head injury resulting from a blow or violent shaking of the brain. May include a period of unconscious or amnesia.

confabulation—A symptom of Korsakoff's syndrome in which the patient supplies ready answers to questions without regard for the truth. The patient who confabulates appears to "fill in" gaps in memory with plausible facts.

conjugate—Working in unison.

constructional apraxia—See apraxia.

construction dyspraxia—Difficulty in reproducing (drawing) simple geometric designs and objects. See apraxia.

contralateral—Referring to the opposite side of the body or brain.

contrecoup—Damage in closed-head injury that is characterized by destruction of brain tissue opposite the site of impact because of the brain's bouncing off the walls of the cranium.

contusion—A form of closed-head injury that produces mild hemorrhaging and associated swelling.

corpus callosum—The brain structure that connects the right and left hemispheres.

cortex—The outer layer of brain tissue comprised of sulci and gyri.

cranial nerves—Twelve pairs of nerves that originate in the brain, and carry sensory and motor signals to and from the periphery of the central nervous system.

cyst—A sac of fluid usually associated with an infectious disorder.

déjà vu—An experience in which new experiences seem familiar and relived. Feelings of déjà vu are common with complex partial seizures.

delirium—An acute, global impairment of cognitive functioning. Delirium is usually reversible, and is most often due to metabolic disturbances of brain function.

dementia—A condition, usually chronic, of global impairment of cognition that occurs in the absence of clouded consciousness. In many cases, such as in Alzheimer's disease, the condition is progressive.

diplopia—Double vision.

dysarthria—Acquired impairment in motor aspects of speech. Dysarthric speech may sound slurred or compressed. Spastic dysarthria, associated with pseudobulbar palsy, is low in pitch and has a raspy sound, with poor articulation. Flaccid dysarthria, associated with bulbar palsy, has an extremely nasal aspect to its sound. Ataxic dysarthria is associated with cerebellar palsy, and produces deficits in articulation and prosody. Hypokinetic dysarthria, found with parkinsonism, results in low-volume speech and less emphasis on accented syllables; there are also articulatory initiation difficulties. Hyperkinetic dysarthria results in prosodic, phonation, and articulatory deficits; the loudness and accents of speech are uncontrolled. There are many disorders that present with combinations of the different types of dysarthria.

dyscalculia—An aphasic symptom characterized by impairment in the ability to appreciate the symbolic significance of numbers and to perform arithmetic calculations.

dysdiadochokinesia—The inability to perform rapid alternating movements. One clinical test for this condition is to have the patient hold out both hands and pronate and supinate them as rapidly as possible.

dysfluency—A disturbance of the fluency of speech.

dysgnosia—In contrast to agnosia, dysgnosia represents a partial, rather than complete, loss of the symbolic significance of information reaching the brain.

dyslexia—See alexia.

dysnomia—See anomia.

dysphagia—Difficulty in swallowing.

dyspnea—Labored breathing.

dyspraxia—See apraxia.

dystonia—Involuntary, slow movements that tend to contort a part of the body for a period. *Dystonic movements* tend to involve large portions of the body, and have a sinuous quality that, when severe, resembles writhing.

edema—Swelling of the brain following cerebral insult or injury. Cerebral edema results from the accumulation of fluid in intercellular tissue.

EEG—Electroencephalographic recording. Known to produce "brain waves." Examination of electrical activity in regions of the brain through the use of electrodes, which measure underlying neuron activity.

embolus—Any foreign object, such as an air bubble or blood clot, which becomes lodged in a vessel or artery, causing an occlusion of blood flow.

encephalitis—Inflammation of the brain.

epilepsy—A condition of abnormal electrical discharges from the brain associated with a temporary alteration in behavior.

ERP—Event-related potentials recording. Examines brief changes of EEG signals in response to discrete sensory signals. See EEG.

eutonia—A general, pervasive feeling of physical well-being.

extrinsic—Outside of the cerebral hemisphere, usually referring to neoplasms or cerebrovascular hemorrhages that are located between the skull and brain.

facial nerve—The seventh cranial nerve. It is involved in the sense of taste, and contains a few other somatic sensory afferent fibers. It is also involved in facial expression. Bell's palsy is the result of compression of the seventh cranial nerve.

fissure—Any deep fold in the cerebral cortex. Fissures define the limits of the cerebral lobes.

flaccid—Relaxed, flabby, or absent muscular tone.

fMRI—Functional magnetic resonance imaging. Permits measurements of regional metabolism of the brain through the examination of high and low use of oxygen. See MRI.

functional—Having a psychiatric or psychological cause.

gait—The particular manner in which a person moves while walking.

general paresis—Tertiary syphilis, characterized by progressive dementia and a generalized paralysis.

glial cells—The connective tissue of the brain (from the Latin word for "glue").

glioma—Any neoplasm arising from glial cells.

glossopharyngeal nerve—The ninth cranial nerve, consisting largely of sensory afferent fibers. Lesions here might result in the loss of the gag reflex and the carotid sinus reflex, as well as loss of the sense of taste and loss of general sensation in the lower third of the tongue.

gyrus—A convolution on the surface of the brain.

hemianopsia—The loss of vision in one-half of a visual field.

hemiballismus—See ballismus.

hemispatial neglect—The failure to detect, report, or orient to one side of the field of experience. Although it is possible with either hemifield, it is more long lasting when it occurs on the left side. It is also known as "hemi-attention" or "unilateral neglect."

hemorrhage—Bleeding.

homonymous hemianopsia—The loss of vision in the same half of the visual field in both eyes.

Huntington's chorea—A genetic abnormality in gene IT-15, chromosome 4, which results in a progressive dementia and includes chorieform movements. Typical onset is between the ages of 35–50. See chorea.

hydrocephalus—Abnormal accumulation of cerebrospinal fluid within the cranium, producing enlarged ventricles and compression of neural tissue.

hypoglossal—The twelfth cranial nerve. It has somatic efferent fibers and serves the tongue. Lesions here will result in lower motor neuron loss and contralateral hemiplegia and ipsilateral paralysis of the tongue.

hypothalamus—A structure dorsal to the thalamus that regulates sleeping, sexual activity, eating, emotions, and other behaviors.

ictal—Related to a seizure (epileptic) episode. For example, cursing is an ictal behavior associated with some forms of temporal lobe epilepsy.

ideational apraxia—See apraxia.

ideomotor apraxia—Sometimes called "ideokinetic apraxia." See apraxia.

idiopathic—A term referring to conditions whose cause is unknown. Epilepsy can be idiopathic or secondary to a known, cerebral insult.

infarct—A region of dead brain tissue associated with an occlusion of the vasculature.

interictal—The period between seizure episodes in an epileptic individual.

intrinsic—Existing within the brain itself.

ipsilateral—On the same side.

ischemia—Any local and temporary deficiency of blood.

jamais vu—An experience associated with some forms of epilepsy, in which familiar surroundings and experiences seem unusual or unreal.

Kayser-Fleischer ring—A brown/green ring around the cornea. This sign is pathognomonic for Wilson's disease.

Korsakoff's syndrome—Deterioration of the brain and cognitive abilities (particularly memory), caused by chronic and severe alcohol abuse and resulting thiamine deficiency.

lesion—Any damage to bodily tissues as a result of disease or injury.

meninges—Three membranes that protect the brain and provide for venous drainage. The dura mater, pia mater, and arachnoid layer comprise the cerebral meninges.

meningioma—A neoplasm arising in the meninges.

meningitis—Inflammation of the meninges, especially of the pia mater and the arachnoid.

metastatic neoplasm—A tumor that develops from abnormal cells that have migrated from another area of the body, most commonly from the lung or breast.

micrographia—Writing with very minute letters or only on a small portion of a page. Sometimes seen in patients with seizure disorders.

mild cognitive impairment—A term used to refer to a constellation of loosely organized symptoms, in which the etiology of these symptoms is unknown.

It has been used to describe the cognitive problems prior to the stage of a progressive dementia, including memory problems without other cognitive impairment, or cognitive difficulty in other areas of functioning with intact memory.

motor impersistence—An inability to continue a motor activity once it is begun, despite commands to do so.

MRI—Magnetic resonance imaging. A large magnet and a radio frequency pulse of a certain resonance generate a signal from the brain to produce an image.

MRS—Magnetic resonance spectroscopy. Varied frequency of radio waves allows for measurements of non-water molecules within the brain. For example, allows for examination of proteins, phospholipids, and cell membranes in the brain.

multiple sclerosis—A disease resulting from degeneration of myelin, characterized by the development of multiple plaques throughout the brain and spinal cord.

mutism—A condition of not speaking. See akinetic mutism.

myelopathy—Disintegration of the myelin sheath. Not to be confused with myopathy.

myoclonus—An abrupt contraction of musculature. Myoclonus results in a jerking motion and ordinarily occurs when a person is falling asleep. Myoclonus in the waking stages may be indicative of neuropathology.

myopathy—Degeneration of muscle fiber. Not to be confused with myelopathy.

myotonia—Delayed relaxation of the muscles. Myotonic dystrophy appears in adulthood and is characterized by an inability of the patient to release a grasp or undo any motor contraction quickly.

myxedema—An endocrine disorder in which there is hypofunction of the thyroid, resulting in psychomotor slowing, apathy, and drowsiness.

neoplasm—Literally "new growth," the term refers to a tumor.

neuralgia—Acute, paroxysmal pain along the course of a nerve.

neuritis—Inflammation of a nerve.

nystagmus—A spasmodic movement of the eyes, either rotary or side to side.

oculomotor nerve—The third cranial nerve. It has efferent fibers to the eye muscles. It is responsible for accommodation and pupil dilation, among other motor activities. Lesions may result in anisocoria, ptosis, or strabismus.

olfactory nerve—The first cranial nerve, serving the sense of smell.

optic nerve—The second cranial nerve, serving the sense of sight.

papilledema—Swelling of the optic disc.

paraphasia—A disturbance in the verbal output of a patient. A literal paraphasia involves the substitution of letters in a word, for example, "ridilicous" for "ridiculous." Semantic or verbal paraphasia involves the substitution of one word for another. The two words are usually in the same semantic class, for example, "shirt" for "pants."

paresthesia—Abnormalities of sensation, especially tactile and somesthetic sensation.

Parkinson's disease—A disorder that primarily affects the motor functions of the cerebellum. Parkinson's disease is characterized by tremors and gait disturbances.

pathognomonic signs—Any sign or symptom that is characteristic of a disease or pathological condition, and that does not occur in the absence of pathology.

PET—Positron emission tomography. Measures metabolic brain activity through the use of an injection of water with unstable radioactive molecules to examine high and low blood flow during a cognitive activity.

Pick's disease—A form of dementia that affects the frontal and temporal lobes, and that is characterized by early loss of social grace and inhibition.

presenile dementia—Severe deterioration of mental functions before the age of 65. Most contemporary investigators minimize the utility of the distinction between presenile and senile dementias.

prosopagnosia—An acquired inability to recognize familiar faces, usually associated with bilateral posterior lesions. (It is different from an inability to recognize unfamiliar faces, which is associated with right posterior lesions.)

pseudodementia—An older term that is used to describe any form of apparent cognitive impairment that is not global and that mimics dementia. A common form is pseudodementia secondary to depression.

ptosis—Permanent dropping of the upper eyelid.

reduplicative paramnesia—A condition whereby the patient has very strong feelings that the current, novel, and unfamiliar environment is actually familiar and personally important. An extremely rare phenomenon.

rigidity—Increased muscle tone that manifests as resistance to passive movement.

scanning speech—Slowed speech with pauses between each syllable.

scotoma—A blind or partially blind area in the visual field.

senile dementia—Severe deterioration of mental functions in persons over the age of 65 years. See dementia.

senile plaques—Areas of incomplete necrosis found in persons with primary neuronal degenerative diseases of the brain. Senile plaques can also be found, in the absence of overt pathology, in most elderly people.

spasm—An involuntary contraction of a muscle group. It can be associated with anxiety or fear, as well as with a neurological disorder.

spasticity—Abnormal increases in muscle tone.

spinal accessory nerve—The eleventh cranial nerve. It has effluent fibers for the branchiomeric musculature. A lesion here might result in paralysis of the trapezium.

stereognosis—The ability to use tactile cues to recognize objects and shapes.

stereotypy—Repetitive movements that serve no purpose.

strabismus—Lack of muscle coordination such that both eyes cannot be directed to the same object.

stroke—A general term used to describe those disorders of the brain that are characterized by disruption of blood flow.

subdural hematoma—A lesion that results from bleeding into the subdural space.

suppression—Any failure to perceive a stimulus on one side of the body with bilateral simultaneous stimulation. Suppressions can exist with auditory, visual, or tactile stimulation. Synonym: extinction.

synapse—The space between the terminal end of an axon and another cell body. Neurotransmitters are released in the synapse and carry signals from one nerve cell to another.

tentorium—The structure that divides the cerebrum from the cerebellum.

thrombus—Any blood clot that forms in an artery or vessel, creating an occlusion. The thrombus typically forms at the bifurcation of a vessel.

tic—Stereotyped movements that may be simple or complex. They are most commonly found in the muscles of the face, and are sensitive to changes in the level of subjective tension.

tinnitus—Ringing in the ears.

transient ischemic attacks (TIAs)—Brief episodes of insufficient blood supply to selected portions of the brain.

tremor—An oscillatory or shaking motion.

trigeminal nerve—The fifth cranial nerve. It has afferent fibers from the face and forehead. It is the conduit for sensation of pain, tactile sensation, and thermal sensation. It also has efferent fibers for the mucous membranes, nose, mouth, teeth, and speech apparatus. It is responsible for the corneal reflex, the tearing reflex, and sneezing.

trochlear nerve—The fourth cranial nerve. It has efferent fibers innervating skeletal muscles. Vertical diplopia is one symptom of a lesion in the trochlear nerve.

unilateral neglect—See hemispatial neglect.

vagus—The tenth cranial nerve. It has an inhibitory effect on heart rate. It has several efferent and afferent fibers to the speech apparatus. Lesions here can result in paralysis of the soft palate, pharynx, and larynx. Possible symptoms include hoarseness, dyspnea, dysphagia, or dysarthria.

ventricles—The spaces within the brain through which cerebrospinal fluid circulates.

vertigo—A sensation of spinning, or the perception that external objects are revolving around an individual. Often used somewhat imprecisely to refer to a feeling of dizziness.

vorbeireden—A verbal response that is incorrect, but that indicates the patient understood the nature of the question, as well as the correct answer.

Wernicke's aphasia—An acquired inability to communicate verbally due to impairment of receptive abilities. Associated with lesions in the posterior portion of the dominant hemisphere.

Wilson's disease—An autosomal recessive genetic disorder of copper metabolism; also known as hepatolenticular degeneration.

witzelsucht—Inappropriate jocularity, most commonly found with right-hemisphere lesions.

References

Adams, R. D., & Victor, M. (1977). *Principles of neurology.* New York: McGraw-Hill.

Al-Khawaja, I., Wade, D. T., & Collins, C. F. (1996). Bedside screening for aphasia: A comparison of two methods. *Journal of Neurology, 243,* 201–204.

Alzheimer's Association. (2009). Retrieved October 10, 2009, from http://www.alz.org

American Heart Association Statistics Committee and Stroke Statistics Subcommittee. (2007). Heart disease and stroke statistics–2007 Update, *Circulation, 115,* e69–e171.

American Psychiatric Association. (1994). *Diagnostic and statistical manual of mental disorders* (4th ed.,). Washington, DC: Author.

American Psychiatric Association. (2000). *Diagnostic and statistical manual of mental disorders* (4th ed., text rev.). Washington, DC: Author.

American Stroke Association. (2009). Retrieved November 1, 2009, from http://www.strokeassociation.org

Armitage, S. B. (1946). An analysis of certain psychological tests used for the evaluation of brain-injury. *Psychological Monographs, 60,* No. 1 (Whole No. 272).

Army Individual Test. (1944). *Manual of directions and scoring.* Washington, DC: War Department, Adjutant General's Office.

Arnett, P. A., & Franzen, M. D. (1997). Performance of substance abusers with memory deficits on measures of malingering. *Archives of Clinical Neuropsychology, 12,* 513–518.

Arnett, P. A., Hammeke, T. A., & Schwartz, L. (1995). Quantitative and qualitative performance on Rey's 15-item test in neurologic patients and dissimulators. *Clinical Neuropsychologist, 9,* 17–26.

Ashendorf, L., Jefferson, A. L., O'Connor, M. K., Chaisson, C., Green, R. C., & Stern, R. A. (2008). Trail making test errors in normal aging, mild cognitive impairment and dementia. *Archives of Clinical Neuropsychology, 23,* 129–137.

Axelrod, B. N., Fichtenberg, N. L., Millis, S. R., & Wertheimer, J. C. (2006). Detecting incomplete effort with digit span from the Wechsler Adult Intelligence Scale-third edition. *Clinical Neuropsychologist, 20,* 513–523.

Babikian, T., Boone, K. B., Lu, P., & Arnold, G. (2006). Sensitivity and specificity of various digit span scores in the detection of suspect effort. *Clinical Neuropsychologist, 20,* 145–159.

Barona, A., Reynolds, C. R., & Chastain, R. (1984). A demographically based index of pre-morbid intelligence for the WAIS-R. *Journal of Consulting and Clinical Psychology, 52,* 885–887.

Barry, P. (1991). *Manual for the Barry rehabilitation inpatient screening of cognition.* Unpublished manuscript. Scottsdale, AZ.

Barry, P., Clark, D. E., Yaguda, M., Higgins, G. E., & Mangel, H. (1989). Rehabilitation inpatient screening of early cognitive recovery. *Archives of Physical Medicine and Rehabilitation, 70,* 902–906.

Baumgartner, C., Pataraia, E., Lindinger, G., & Deeke, L. (2000). Neuromagnetic recordings in temporal lobe epilepsy. *Journal of Clinical Neurophysiology, 17,* 177–189.

Beaumont, J. G., & Davidoff, J. B. (1992). Assessment of visuo-perceptual dysfunction. In J. R. Crawford, D. M. Parker, & W. W. McKinlay (Eds.), *A handbook of neuropsychological assessment.* Hove, UK: Lawrence Erlbaum.

Bechara, A., Damasio, A. R., Damasio, H., & Anderson, S. W. (1994). Insensitivity to future consequences following damage to human prefrontal cortex. *Cognition, 50,* 7–15.

Belanger, H. G., Vanderploeg, R. D., Curtiss, G., & Warden, D. L. (2007). Recent neuroimaging techniques in mild traumatic brain injury. *Journal of Neuropsychiatry and Clinical Neurosciences, 19,* 5–20.

Benedict, R. H. (1997). *Brief Visuospatial Memory Test–Revised: Professional manual.* Odessa, FL: Psychological Assessment Resources.

Benedict, R. H. B., & Zgaljardic, D. J. (1998). Practice effects during repeated administrations of memory tests with and without alternate forms. *Journal of Clinical and Experimental Neuropsychology, 20,* 339–352.

Bender, L. A. (1938). A visual motor gestalt test and its clinical use. *American Orthopsychiatric Association Research Monographs, 3.*

Benton, A. L. (1968). Differential behavioral effects in frontal lobe disease. *Neuropsychologia, 6,* 53–60.

Benton, A. L. (1974). *The revised visual retention test* (4th ed.). New York: Psychological Corporation.

Benton, A. L. (1994). Neuropsychological assessment. *Annual Reviews of Psychology, 45,* 1–23.

Benton, A. L., Hamsher, K. deS., Varney, N. R., & Spreen, O. (1983). *Contributions to neuropsychological assessment.* New York: Oxford University Press.

Benton, A. L., Sivan, A. B., Hamsher, K. DeS., Varney, N. R., & Spreen, O. (1994). *Contributions to neuropsychological assessment* (2nd ed.). New York: Oxford University Press.

Benton, A. L., & Van Allen, M. W. (1968). Impairment in facial recognition in patients with cerebral disease. *Cortex, 4,* 344–358.

Benton, A. L., Van Allen, M. W., & Fogel, M. L. (1964). Temporal orientation in cerebral disease. *Journal of Nervous and Mental Disease, 139,* 110–119.

Berg, E. A. (1948). A simple objective technique for measuring flexibility in thinking. *Journal of General Psychology, 39,* 15–22.

Berger, G., Frolich, L., Weber, B., & Pantel, J. (2008). Diagnostic accuracy of the clock drawing test: The relevance of "time setting" in screening for dementia. *Journal of Geriatric Psychiatry and Neurology, 21*(4), 250–260.

Bernard, L. C. (1990). Prospects for faking believable memory deficits on neuropsychological tests and the use of incentives in simulation research. *Journal of Clinical and Experimental Neuropsychology, 12,* 715–728.

Bernard, L. C. (1991). The detection of faked deficits on the Rey Auditory Verbal Learning Test: The effect of serial position. *Archives of Clinical Neuropsychology, 6*, 81–88.

Bernat, J. L. (2009). Ethical issues in the treatment of severe brain injury: The impact of new technologies. In N. D. Schiff & S. Laureys (Eds.), Disorders of consciousness. *Annals of the New York Academy of Science* (pp. 117–130). New York: Wiley-Blackwell.

Biederman, J., Mick, F., & Faraone, S. V. (2000). Age-dependent decline of symptoms of attention deficit hyperactivity disorder: Impact of remission definition and symptom type. *American Journal of Psychiatry, 157*, 816–818.

Billingslea, F. Y. (1963). The Bender-gestalt: A review and a perspective. *Psychological Bulletin, 60*, 233–251.

Blanchard, J. J., & Neale, J. M. (1994). The neuropsychological signature of schizophrenia: Generalized or differential deficit? *American Journal of Psychiatry, 151*, 40–48.

Boller, F., & Vignolo, L. A. (1966). Latent sensory aphasia in hemisphere-damaged patients: An experimental study with the token test. *Brain, 89*, 815–831.

Bond, M. R. (1986). Neurobehavioral sequelae of closed head injury. In L. Grant & K. M. Adams (Eds.), *Neuropsychological assessment of neuropsychiatric disorders* (pp. 347–373). New York: Oxford University Press.

Boone, K. B., Lu, P., & Wen, J. (2005). Comparison of various RAVLT scores in the detection of noncredible memory performance. *Archives of Clinical Neuropsychology, 20*, 301–319.

Bornstein, R. A. (1991). Report of the Division 40 Task Force on Education, Accreditation and Credentialing: Recommendations for education and training of nondoctoral personnel in clinical neuropsychology. *Clinical Neuropsychologist, 5*, 20–23.

Borowski, J. G., Benton, A. L., & Spreen, O. (1967). Word fluency and brain damage. *Neuropsychologia, 5*, 135–140.

Brandt, J., & Benedict, R. H. B. (2001). *Hopkins Verbal Learning Test–Revised. Professional manual*. Lutz, FL: Psychological Assessment Resources.

Bresnahan, M., Begg, M. D., Brown, A., Schaefer, C., Sohler, N., Insel, B., et al. (2007). Race and risk of schizophrenia in a US birth cohort: Another example of health disparity? *International Journal of Epidemiology, 36*, 751–758.

Brilliant, P. J., & Gynther, M. D. (1963). Relationships between performance on three tests for organicity and selected patient variables. *Journal of Consulting Psychology, 27*, 474–479.

Browne, T. R., & Holmes, G. L. (2004). *Handbook of epilepsy* (3rd ed.). Philadelphia: Lippincott, Williams and Wilkins.

Brugnolo, A., Nobili, F., Barbieri, M. B., Dessi, B., Ferro, A., Girtler, N., et al. (2009). The factorial structure of the mini mental state examination (MMSE) in Alzheimer's disease. *Archives of Gerontology and Geriatrics, 49*, 180–185.

Bubb, D. I. (1984). *Neurologic problems*. Oradell, NJ: Medical Economics Books.

Buschke, H. (1973). Selective reminding for analysis of memory and learning. *Journal of Verbal Learning and Verbal Behavior, 12*, 543–550.

Buschke, H., & Fuld, P. A. (1974). Evaluating storage, retention, and retrieval in disordered memory and learning. *Neurology, 24*, 1019–1025.

Butcher, J. N., Dahlstrom, W. G., Graham, J. R., Tellegen, A., & Kaemmer, B. (1989). *The Minnesota Multiphasic Personality Inventory-2 (MMPI-2). Manual for administration and scoring.* Minneapolis, MN, University of Minnesota Press.

Butters, N., Grant, I., Haxby, J., Judd, L. L., Martin, A., McClelland, J., et al. (1990). Assessment of AIDS-related cognitive changes: Recommendations of the NIMH Workgroup on neuro-psychological assessment approaches. *Journal of Clinical and Experimental Neuropsychology, 12*, 963–978.

Canter, A. (1966). A background interference procedure to increase sensitivity of the Bender-gestalt test to organic brain damage. *Journal of Consulting Psychology, 30*, 91–95.

Centers for Disease Control. (2001). The global HIV/AIDS epidemic, 2001. *Morbidity and Mortality Weekly Report, 50.*

Chelune, G. J., & Baer, R. A. (1986). Developmental norms for the Wisconsin Card Sorting Test. *Journal of Clinical and Experimental Neuropsychology, 8*, 219–228.

Chiaravalloti, N. D., Balzano, J., Moore, N. B., & Deluca, J. (2009). The open-trial selective reminding test. *Clinical Neuropsychologist, 23*(2), 231–254.

Choca, J., Laatsch, L., Garside, D., & Arnemann, C. (1987). *Category test computer program 6.0.* Tonowanda, NY: MHS.

CogState, Ltd. (1999). *CogSport.* Parville, Victoria, Australia: Author.

Cohen, M. J., & Stanczak, D. E. (2000). On the reliability, validity, and cognitive structure of the Thurstone word fluency test. *Archives of Clinical Neuropsychology, 15*, 267–279.

Costa, L. D. (1975). The relation of visuospatial dysfunction to digit span performance in patients with cerebral lesions. *Cortex, 11*, 31–36.

Costa, L. D., Vaughan, H. G., Levita, E., & Farber, N. (1963). Purdue pegboard as a predictor of the presence and laterality of cerebral lesions. *Journal of Consulting Psychology, 27*, 133–137.

Costello, S. D., Bieliauskas, L. A., & Terpenning, M. (1992, August). *The sensitivity of neuropsychological screening instruments: A comparison of the MMSE and the NCSE.* Paper presented at the annual meeting of the American Psychological Association, Washington, DC.

Crawford, J. R. (1992). Current and premorbid intelligence measures in neuropsychological assessment. In J. R. Crawford, D. M. Parker, & W. W. McKinlay (Eds.), *A handbook of neuropsychological assessment.* East Sussex, UK: Lawrence Erlbaum.

Crow, R. R. (1982). Recent genetic research in schizophrenia. In F. A. Henn & H. A. Nasrallah (Eds.), *Schizophrenia as a brain disease* (pp. 40–55). New York: Oxford University Press.

Cruice, M. N., & Worrall, L. E. (2000). Boston Naming Test results for healthy older Australians: A longitudinal and cross-sectional study. *Aphasiology, 14*, 143–155.

Crum, R. M., Anthony, J. C., Bassett, S. S., & Folstein, M. F. (1993). Population-based norms for the Mini-Mental State Examination by age and education level. *Journal of the American Medical Association, 269*(18), 2386–2391.

Cummings, J. L. (1985). *Clinical neuropsychiatry.* Orlando, FL: Grune & Stratton.

Curtis, K. L., Greve, K. W., Bianchini, K J., & Brennan, A. (2006). California Verbal Learning Test indicators of malingered neurocognitive dysfunction sensitivity and specificity in traumatic brain injury. *Assessment, 13*, 46–61.

Dal Canto, M. C. (1989). AIDS and the nervous system. *Human Pathology, 20*, 410–416.
Davies, A. (1968). The influence of age on trail making test performance. *Journal of Clinical Psychology, 24*, 96–98.
DeJager, C. A., Schrinemaekaers, A. C. M. C., Honey, T. E. M., & Budge, M. M. (2009). Detection of MCI in the clinic: Evaluation of the sensitivity and specificity of a computerized test battery, the Hopkins verbal learning test and the MMSE. *Age and Ageing, 38*, 455–460.
Delaney, R. C., Prevey, M. L., Cramer, J., & Mattson, R. H. (1992). Test-retest comparability and control subject data for the Rey-auditory verbal learning test and Rey-Osterrieth/Taylor complex figures. *Archives of Clinical Neuropsychology, 7*(6), 523–528.
Delis, D., Kaplan, E., & Kramer, J. (2001). *The Delis-Kaplan executive functions system.* San Antonio, TX: Psychological Corporation.
DeRenzi, E., Faglioni, R., Savoiardo, M., & Vignolo, L. A. (1966). The influence of aphasia and of the hemisphere side of the cerebral lesion on abstract thinking. *Cortex, 2*, 399–420.
DeRenzi, E., & Spinnler, H. (1967). Visual recognition in patients with unilateral cerebral disease. *Journal of Nervous and Mental Disease, 142*, 515–525.
DeRenzi, E., & Vignolo, L. A. (1962). The token test: A sensitive test to detect disturbances in aphasics. *Brain, 85*, 665–678.
Diamond, A. (2007). Consequences of variations in genes that affect dopamine in prefrontal cortex. *Cerebral Cortex, 17*, 161–170.
Djaldetti, R., Treves, T. A., Ziv, I., Melamed, E., Lampl, Y., & Lorberboym, M. (2009). Use of a single [(123)I]-FP-CIT SPECT to predict the severity of clinical symptoms of Parkinson disease. *Neurological Sciences, 30*, 301–305.
Donders, J. (1998). Validity of the Kaufman Short Neuropsychological Assessment Procedure (KSNAP). *International Journal of Neuroscience, 94*, 275–286.
Duffy, F. H. (1981). Brain electrical activity mapping (BEAM): Computerized access to complex brain function. *International Journal of Neuroscience, 13*, 55–65.
Duffy, F. H. (1982). Topographic display of evoked potentials: Clinical applications of brain electrical activity mapping (BEAM). *Annals of the New York Academy of Science, 388*, 183–196.
Duffy, F. H., Albert, M. S., & McAnulty, G. (1984). Brain electrical activity in patients with presenile and senile dementia of the Alzheimer's type. *Annals of Neurology, 16*, 439–448.
Dujardin, K., Defebvre, L., Grunberg, C., Becquet, E., & Destée, A. (2004). Memory and executive function in sporadic and familial Parkinson's disease. *Brain, 124*, 389–398.
Dunn, L. M., & Dunn, D. M. (2007). *Peabody Picture Vocabulary Test* (4th ed.). Circle Pines, MN: American Guidance Service.
Dvorine, I. (1953). *Dvorine pseudo-isochromatic plates* (2nd ed.). Baltimore, MD: Waverly Press.
Eberwein, C. A., Pratt, S. R., McNeil, M. R., Fossett, T. R. D., Szuminsky, N. J., & Doyle, P. J. (2007). Auditory performance characteristics of the Computerized Revised Token Test (CRTT). *Journal of Speech, Language, and Hearing Research, 50*, 865–877.

Eisenberger, N. I., Lieberman, M. D., & Williams, K. D. (2003). Does rejection hurt? An fMRI study of social exclusion. *Science, 302,* 290–292.
Eisenson, J. (1973). *Adult aphasia.* New York: Appleton-Century-Crofts.
Ekstrom, R. B., French, J. W., Harman, H. H., & Dermen, D. (1976). *Manual for kit of factor-referenced cognitive tests.* Princeton, NJ: Educational Testing Service.
Ellingsen, D. G., Lorentzen, P., & Langard, S. (1997). A neuropsychological study of patients exposed to organic solvents. *International Journal of Occupational and Environmental Health, 3,* 177–183.
Elwood, D. L., & Griffin, R. (1972). Individual intelligence testing without the examiner. *Journal of Consulting and Clinical Psychology, 38,* 9–14.
Enderby, P., & Crow, E. (1996). Frenchay Aphasia Screening Test: Validity and screening. *Disability and Rehabilitation, 18*(5), 238–240.
Engel, J., Jr. (2001). A proposed diagnostic scheme for people with epileptic seizures and with epilepsy: Report of the ILAE Task Force on Classification and Terminology. *Epilepsia., 42,* 796–803.
Erickson, R. C., Calsyn, D. A., & Scheupbach, C. S. (1978). Abbreviating the Halstead-Reitan neuropsychological test battery. *Journal of Clinical Psychology, 34,* 922–926.
Erlanger, D. M., Feldman, D., & Kutner, K. (1999). *Concussion resolution index.* New York: HeadMinder, Inc.
Etherton, J. L., Bianchini, K. J., Greve, K. W., & Heinly, M. T. (2005). Sensitivity and specificity of reliable digit span in malingered pain-related disability. *Assessment, 12,* 130–136.
Fama, R., Sullivan, E. V., Shear, P. K., Cahn-Weiner, D. A., Yesavage, J. A., Tinklinberg, J. R., et al. (1998). Fluency performance patterns in Alzheimer's disease and Parkinson's disease. *Clinical Neuropsychologist, 12,* 487–499.
Feldman, R. G., Ricks, N. L., & Baker, E. L. (1980). Neuropsychological effects of industrial toxins: A review. *American Journal of Industrial Medicine, 1,* 211–227.
Feldstein, S. N., Keller, F. R., Portman, R. E., Durham, R. L., Klebe, K. J., & Davis, H. P. (1999). A comparison of the computerized and standard versions of the Wisconsin card sorting test. *Clinical Neuropsychology, 13,* 303–313.
Fields, R. B., Starratt, C., Fishman, E., Cisewski, D., & Coffey, C. E. (1993). Detecting change in cognitive status following treatment for organic mood disorder: MMSE vs. NCSE. *Archives of Clinical Neuropsychology, 8,* 223.
Fisher, H. L., & Rose, D. (2005). Comparison of the effectiveness of two versions of the Rey Memory Test in discriminating between actual and simulated memory impairment, with and without the addition of a standard memory test. *Journal of Clinical and Experimental Neuropsychology, 27,* 840–858.
Flor-Henry, P. (1976). Lateralized temporal-limbic dysfunction and psychopathology. *Annals of the New York Academy of Science, 286,* 779–795.
Fogel, M. L. (1965). The proverbs test in the appraisal of cerebral disease. *Journal of General Psychology, 72,* 269–275.
Folstein, M. E., Folstein, S. E., & McHugh, P. R. (1975). "Mini-Mental State": A practical method for grading the cognitive state of patients for the clinician. *Journal of Psychiatric Research, 12,* 189–198.
Fowler, K. S., Saling, M. M., Conway, E. L., Semple, J. M., & Louis, W. J. (2002). Paired associate performance in the early detection of DAT. *Journal of the International Neuropsychological Society, 8,* 58–71.

Frederick, R. I., & Foster, H. G. (1991). Multiple measures of malingering on a forced-choice test of cognitive ability. *Psychological Assessment, 3,* 596–602.
Frederick, R. I., Sarfaty, S. D., Johnston, J. D., & Powel, J. (1994). Validation of a detector of response bias on a forced-choice test of nonverbal ability. *Neuropsychology, 8,* 118–125.
Frederick, R. I., & Speed, F. M. (2007). On the interpretation of below-chance responding in forced-choice tests. *Assessment, 14,* 3–11.
French, C. C., & Beaumont, J. G. (1987). The reaction of psychiatric patients to computerized assessment. *British Journal of Clinical Psychology, 26,* 267–277.
Fukui, H., Murai, T., Fukuyama, H., Hayashi, T., & Hanakawa, T. (2005). Functional activity related to risk anticipation during performance of the Iowa Gambling Task. *Neuroimage, 24,* 253–259.
Gale, S. D., & Hopkins, R. O. (2004). Effects of hypoxia on the brain: Neuroimaging and neuropsychological findings following carbon monoxide poisoning and obstructive sleep apnea. *Journal of the International Neuropsychological Society, 10,* 60–71.
Galletly, C. A., Clark, C. R., McFarlane, A. C., & Weber, D. L. (2001). Working memory in posttraumatic stress disorder—An event-related potential study. *Journal of Traumatic Stress, 14,* 295–309.
Gates, A. I., & MacGinitie, W. H. (1969). *Gates-MacGinitie reading tests.* New York: Teachers College Press.
Geffen, G., Hoar, K. J., O'Hanlon, A. P., Clark, C. R., & Geffen, L. B. (1990). Performance measures of 16- to 86-year-old males and females on the auditory verbal learning test. *Clinical Neuropsychologist, 4,* 45–63.
Golden, C. J. (1976). The identification of brain damage by an abbreviated form of the Halstead-Reitan neuropsychological battery. *Journal of Clinical Psychology, 32,* 821–826.
Golden, C. J. (1978). *The Stroop Color and Word Test: A manual for clinical and experimental uses.* Chicago: Stoelting.
Golden, C. J. (1979). *Clinical interpretation of objective psychological tests.* New York: Grune & Stratton.
Golden, C. (2004). The Adult Luria Nebraska Neuropsychological battery. In M. Hersen (Ed.), *Comprehensive handbook of psychological assessment* (pp. 133–146). New York: Wiley.
Golden, C. J. (1981). *Diagnosis and rehabilitation in clinical neuropsychology* (2nd ed.). Springfield, IL: Charles C Thomas.
Golden, C. J., Hammeke, T. A., & Purisch, A. D. (1985). *The Luria-Nebraska neuropsychological battery.* Los Angeles: Western Psychological Services.
Golding, E. (1989). *The Middlesex elderly assessment of mental state.* Fareham, UK: Thames Valley Test Company.
Goldstein, K., & Scheerer, M. (1941). Abstract and concrete behavior: An experimental study with special tests. *Psychological Monographs, 239.*
Gollin, E. S. (1960). Developmental studies of visual recognition of incomplete objects. *Perceptual and Motor Skills, 11,* 289–298.
Gontkovsky, S. T., & Souheaver, G. T. (2000). Are brain-damaged patients inappropriately labeled as malingering using the 21-item Test and the WMS-R Logical Memory Forced Choice Recognition Test? *Psychological Reports, 87,* 512–514.

Gonzalez, E. A., Dieter, J. N. I., Natale, R. A., & Tanner, S. L. (2001). Neuropsychological evaluation of higher functioning homeless persons: A comparison of an abbreviated test battery to the Mini-Mental State Exam. *Journal of Nervous and Mental Disease, 189,* 176–181.

Goodglass, H., Kaplan E. F., & Weintraub, S. (2001). *The Boston Naming Test* (2nd ed.). Philadelphia: Lippincott, Williams & Wilkins.

Gorham, D. R. (1956). A proverbs test for clinical and experimental use. *Psychological Reports, 2*(Suppl. 1), 1–12.

Grant, D. A., & Berg, E. A. (1948). A behavioral analysis of degree of reinforcement and ease of shifting to new responses in a Weigl-type card-sorting problem. *Journal of Experimental Psychology, 38,* 401–411.

Green, P. (2007). Making comparisons between forced-choice effort tests. In K. B. Boone (Ed.), *Assessment of feigned cognitive impairment* (pp. 50-77). New York: Guilford.

Greene, J. D., & Paxton, J. M. (2009). Patterns of neural activity associated with honest and dishonest moral decisions. *Proceedings of the National Academy of Sciences of the United States of America, 106*(30), 12506–12511.

Greve, K. W., Ord, J., Curtis, K. L., Bianchini, K. J., & Brennan, A. (2008). Detecting malingering in traumatic brain injury and chronic pain: A comparison of three forced-choice symptom validity tests. *Clinical Neuropsychologist, 22,* 896–918.

Greve, K. W., Springer, S., Bianchini, K. J., Black, F. W., Heinly, M. T., Love, J. M., et al. (2007). Malingering in toxic exposure: Classification accuracy of reliable digit span and WAIS-III Digit Span scaled scores. *Assessment, 14,* 12–21.

Greiffenstein, M. F., Greve, K. W., Bianchini, K. J., & Baker, W. J. (2008). Test of Memory Malingering and Word Memory Test: A new comparison of failure concordance rates. *Archives of Clinical Neuropsychology, 23,* 801–807.

Gur, R. C., Ragland, J. D., & Moberg, P. J., (2001). Computerized neurocognitive scanning: I. Methodology and validation in healthy people. *Neuropsychopharmacology, 25,* 766–776.

Hain, J. D. (1964). The Bender-gestalt test: A scoring method for identifying brain damage. *Journal of Consulting Psychology, 28,* 34–40.

Hall, R. C. W. (1980). Depression. In R. C. W. Hall (Ed.), *Psychiatric presentations of medical illness: Somatopsychic disorders* (pp. 37–63). New York: SP Medical & Scientific Books.

Halstead, W. C. (1947). *Brain and intelligence.* Chicago: University of Chicago Press.

Halstead, W. C., & Wepman, J. M. (1949). The Halstead-Wepman aphasia screening test. *Journal of Speech and Hearing Disorders, 14,* 9–15.

Hamberger, M. J., Goodman, R. R., Perrine, K., & Tamny, T. (2001). Anatomic dissociation of auditory and visual naming in the lateral temporal cortex. *Neurology, 56,* 56–61.

Hannay, J. H. (1986). *Experimental techniques in human neuropsychology.* New York: Oxford University Press.

Hannay, J. H., & Levin, H. S. (1985). Selective reminding test: An examination of the equivalence of four forms. *Journal of Clinical and Experimental Neuropsychology, 7,* 251–263.

Hannay, H. J., Bieliauskas, L., Crosson, A. A., Hammeke, T. A., Hamsher, de K. S., & Koffler, S. (Eds.). (1998). Proceedings of the Houston Conference on Specialty

Education and Training in Clinical Neuropsychology. *Archives of Clinical Neuropsychology, 13,* 157–250.

Hart, R. P., Kwentus, J. A., Taylor, J. R., & Hamer, R. M. (1988). Productive naming and memory in depression and Alzheimer's type dementia. *Archives of Clinical Neuropsychology, 3,* 313–322.

Hartje, W., Kerschensteiner, M., Poeck, K., & Argass, B. (1973). A cross-validation study on the token test. *Neuropsychologia, 11,* 119–121.

Heaton, R. K. (1981). *Manual for the Wisconsin Card Sorting Test.* Odessa, FL: Psychological Assessment Resources.

Heaton, R. K. (1999). *Wisconsin card sorting test: Computer version 3 for Windows®* (research ed.). Lutz, FL: Psychological Assessment Resources.

Heaton, R. K., Avitable, N., Grant, I., & Matthews, C. G. (1999). Further cross validation of regression-based neuropsychological norms with an update for the Boston Naming Test. *Journal of Clinical and Experimental Neuropsychology, 21,* 572–582.

Heaton, R. K., Grant, I., Butters, N., White, D. A., Kirson, D., Atkinson, J. H., et al. (1995). The HNRC 500–Neuropsychology of HIV infection at different disease stages. HIV Neurobehavioral Research Center. *Journal of the International Neuropsychological Society, 1,* 231–251.

Heimburger, R. F., & Reitan, R. M. (1961). Easily administered written test for lateralizing brain lesions. *Journal of Neurosurgery, 18,* 301–312.

Henn, R. A., & Nasrallah, H. A. (1982). *Schizophrenia as a brain disease.* New York: Oxford University Press.

Ho, D., Bredesen, D. E., Vinters, H. V., & Daar, E. S. (1989). AIDS dementia complex. *Annals of Internal Medicine, 11,* 400–409.

Hutt, M. (1969). *The Hutt adaptation of the Bender-gestalt test* (2nd ed.). New York: Grune & Stratton.

Ishihara, S. (1983). *Ishihara's Test for Color Blindness.* Tokyo: Kanehara Shuppan.

Iverson, G. L., & Franzen, M. D. (1996). Using multiple objective memory procedures to detect simulated malingering. *Journal of Clinical and Experimental Neuropsychology, 18,* 38–51.

Iverson, G. L., Franzen, M. D., & McCracken, L. M. (1991). Evaluation of an objective assessment technique for the detection of malingered memory deficits. *Law and Human Behavior, 15,* 667–676.

Iverson, G. L., Franzen, M. D., & McCracken, L. M. (1994). Application of a forced-choice memory procedure designed to detect experimental malingering. *Archives of Clinical Neuropsychology, 9,* 437–450.

Iverson, G. L., Williamson, D. J., Ropacki, M., & Reilly, K. J. (2007). Frequency of abnormal scores on the neuropsychological assessment battery screening module (S-NAB) in a mixed neurological sample. *Applied Neuropsychology, 14*(3), 178–182.

Ivnik, R. J., Malec, J. F., & Smith, G. E. (1996). Neuropsychological tests' norms above age 55: COWAT, BNT, MAE token, WRAT-R reading, AMNART, STROOP, TMT, and JLO. *Clinical Neuropsychologist, 10,* 262–278.

Jacobs, J. W., Bernhard, M. R., Delgado, A., & Strain, J. J. (1977). Screening for organic mental syndromes in the medically ill. *Annals of Internal Medicine, 86,* 40–46.

Jager, T. E., Weiss, H. B., Coben, J. H., & Pepe, P. E. (2000). Traumatic brain injuries evaluated in U.S. emergency departments, 1992–1994. *Academic Emergency Medicine, 7,* 134–140.

Johnson, J. E., Hellkamp, D. T., & Lottman, T. J. (1971). The relationship between intelligence, brain damage, and Hutt-Briskin errors on the Bender-Gestalt. *Journal of Clinical Psychology, 27*, 84–88.

Jurica, P. J., Leitten, C. L., & Mattis, S. (2001). *Dementia rating scale-2 (DRS-2) professional manual.* Odessa, FL: Psychological Assessment Resources.

Kaemingk, K. L., & Kazniak, A. W. (1989). Neuropsychological aspects of human immunodeficiency virus infection. *Clinical Neuropsychologist, 3*, 309–326.

Kaplan, E., Goodglass, H., & Weintraub, S. (1983). *Boston Naming Test.* Philadelphia: Lea & Febiger.

Kaplan E. F., Goodglass, H., & Weintraub, S. (2001). *The Boston Naming Test* (2nd ed.). Philadelphia: Lippincott, Williams & Wilkins.

Kaufman, A., & Kaufman, N. (1994). *Kaufman short neuropsychological procedure.* Circle Pines, MN: American Guidance Service.

Kiernan, R. J., Mueller, J., Langston, J. W., & van Dyke, C. (1987). The neurobehavioral cognitive status examination: A brief but differentiated approach to assessment. *Annals of Internal Medicine, 107*, 481–485.

Kilpatrick, B., & Hall, R. (1980). Seizure disorders. In C. W. Hall (Ed.), *Psychiatric presentations of medical illness* (pp. 243–258). New York: Spectrum Publications.

Kim, Y. S., Lee, K. M., Choi, B. H., Sohn, E. H., & Lee, A. Y. (2009). Relation between the clock drawing tests (CDT) and structural changes of brain in dementia. *Archives of Gerontology and Geriatrics, 48*, 218–221.

King, J. H., Gfeller, J. D., & Davis, H. P. (1998). Detecting simulated memory impairment with the Rey Auditory Verbal Learning Test: Implications of base rates and study generalizability. *Journal of Clinical and Experimental Neuropsychology, 20*, 603–612.

Kinsbourne, M., & Warrington, E. K. (1962). A study of finger agnosia. *Brain, 85*, 47–66.

Knehr, C. A. (1965). Revised approach to detection of cerebral damage: Progressive matrices revisited. *Psychological Reports, 17*, 71–77.

Knight, J. A., Pimental, R. A., Miller, S., & McWilliams, J. (1990, August). *Use of the mini-inventory of right brain injury (MIRBI) in psychiatric samples.* Paper presented at the annual meeting of the American Psychological Association, Boston, MA.

Koch, S. Forteza, A., Lavernia, C., Romano, J. G., Campo-Bustillo, I., Campo, N., et al. (2007). Cerebral fat microembolism and cognitive decline after hip and knee replacement. *Stroke, 38*, 1079.

Kurtzke, J. F., & Wallin, M. T. (2000). Epidemiology. In J. S. Burks & K. P. Johnson (Eds.), *Multiple sclerosis: Diagnosis, medical management and rehabilitation.* New York: Demos Medical.

Laukka, E. J., Jones, S., Fratiglioni, L., & Backman, L. (2004). Cognitive functioning in preclinical dementia: A 6 year follow-up. *Stroke, 35*, 1805–1809.

Lechtenberg, R. (1982). *The psychiatrist's guide to diseases of the nervous system.* New York: John Wiley.

Leskin, L. P., & White, P. M. (2007). Attentional networks reveal executive function deficits in posttraumatic stress disorder. *Neuropsychology, 21*, 275–284.

Levin, H. S., & Benton, A. L. (1975). Temporal orientation in patients with brain disease. *Applied Neurophysiology, 38*, 56–60.

Levin, H. S., O'Donnell, V. M., & Grossman, R. G. (1979). The Galveston Orientation and Amnesia Test: A practical scale to assess cognition after head injury. *Journal of Nervous and Mental Disease, 167*, 675–684.

Levine, J., & Feirstein, A. (1972). Differences in test performance between brain damaged, schizophrenic, and medical patients. *Journal of Consulting and Clinical Psychology, 39,* 508–520.

Lezak, M. D., Howieson, D. B., & Loring, D. (2004). *Neuropsychological assessment* (4th ed.). New York: Oxford University Press.

Lishman, W. A. (1978). *Organic psychiatry: The psychological consequences of cerebral disorder.* London: Blackwell Scientific.

Lopez, M. N., Charter, R. A., Mostafavi, B., Nibut, L. P., & Smith, W. E. (2005). Psychometric properties of the Folstein Mini-Mental State examination. *Archives of Clinical Neuropsychology, 21,* 7, 677–686.

Lovell, M. R., Collins, M. W., Podell, K., Powell, J., & Maroon, J. (2000). *ImPACT: Immediate post-concussion assessment and cognitive testing.* Pittsburgh, PA: Neuro-Health Systems, LLC.

Luciana, M. (2003). Practitioner review: Computerised assessment of neuro-psychological function in children: Clinical and research applications of the Cambridge Neuropsychological Testing Automated Battery (CANTAB). *Journal of Child Psychology and Psychiatry and Allied Disciplines, 44,* 1–15.

Macaulay, C., Battista, M., Lebby, P. C., & Mueller, J. (2003). Geriatric performance on the Neurobehavioral Cognitive Status Examination (Cognistat): What is normal? *Archives of Clinical Neuropsychology, 18,* 463–471.

Maschke, M., Kastrup, O., Esser, S., Ross, B., Hengge, U., & Hufnagel, A. (2000). Incidence and prevalence of neurological disorders associated with HIV since the introduction of highly active antiretroviral therapy (HAART). *Journal of Neurology, Neurosurgery and Psychiatry, 69,* 376–380.

MacGinitie, W. H., MacGinitie, R. K., Maria, K., & Dreyer, L. G. (2000). *Gates-MacGinitie Reading Tests* (4th ed.). Itasca, IL: Riverside.

Maj, M. (1990). Psychiatric aspects of HIV-1 infection and AIDS. *Psychological Medicine, 20,* 547–563.

Marchand, Y., D'Arcy, R. C. N., & Connolly, J. F. (2002). Linking neurophysiological and neuropsychological measures for aphasia assessment. *Clinical Neurophysiology, 113,* 1715–1722.

Maschke, M., Kastrup, O., Esser, S., Ross, B., Hengge, U., & Huffnagel, A. (2000). Incidence and prevalence of neurological disorders associated with HIV since the introduction of highly active antiretroviral therapy (HAART). *Journal of Neurology, Neurosurgery, and Psychiatry, 69,* 376–380.

Matarazzo, J. D. (1990). Psychological assessment versus psychological testing: Validation from Binet to the school, clinic, and courtroom. *American Psychologist, 45,* 999–1017.

Mather, N., & Woodcock, R. W. (2001). *Woodcock-Johnson III tests of cognitive abilities. Examiner's manual.* Itasca, IL: Riverside.

Mattis, S. (1976). Mental status examination for organic mental syndrome in the elderly patient. In L. Bellak & T. B. Karasu (Eds.), *Geriatric psychiatry.* New York: Grune & Stratton.

Mattis, S. N. (1988). *Dementia rating scale.* Odessa, FL: Psychological Assessment Resources.

McFie, J. (1960). Psychological testing in clinical neurology. *Journal of Nervous and Mental Disease, 131,* 383–393.

McFie, J. (1975). *Assessment of organic intellectual impairment.* New York: Academic Press.

McNamara, K. M., Wechsler, F. S., & Munger, M. P. (1984, August). *The Halstead-Reitan versus an abbreviated battery: Feasibility and imitations.* Paper presented at the annual convention of the American Psychological Association, Toronto, ON, Canada.

McNeil, M., & Prescott, T. (1978). *Revised token test.* Austin, TX: Pro Ed.

Meyers, J. E., & Rohling, M. L. (2004). Validation of the Meyers short battery on mild TBI patients. *Archives of Clinical Neuropsychology, 19,* 637–651.

Milberg, W. P., Hebben, N., & Kaplan, E. (2009). The Boston Process Approach to neuropsychological assessment (3rd ed., pp. 42–65). In I. Grant & K. M. Adams (Eds.), *Neuropsychological assessment of neuropsychiatric and neuromedical disorders.* New York: Oxford University Press.

Miller, D. H. (2003). Magnetic resonance imaging in multiple sclerosis: An overview. In J. A. Cohen & R. Rudick (Eds.), *Multiple sclerosis therapeutics* (2nd ed.). New York: Martin Dunitz.

Milner, B. (1962). Laterality effects in audition. In V. B. Mountcastle (Ed.), *Interhemispheric relations and cerebral dominance* (pp. 143–169). Baltimore, MD: Johns Hopkins University Press.

Milner, B. (1967). Brain mechanisms suggested by studies of temporal lobes. In C. H. Millikan & F. L. Darley (Eds.), *Brain mechanisms underlying speech and language* (pp. 25–47). New York: Grune & Stratton.

Mitrushina, M., Boone, K. B., Razani, J., & D'Elia, L. F. (1999). *Handbook of normative data for neuropsychological assessment* (2nd ed.). New York: Oxford University Press.

Mooney, C. M., & Ferguson, G. A. (1951). A new closure test. *Canadian Journal of Psychology, 5,* 129–133.

Moore, K. R., Funke, M. E., Constantino, C., Katzman, G. L., & Lewine, J. D. (2002). Integration of MEG and high-resolution surface-coil MR imaging improves the identification of epileptogenic lesions in patients with neocortical epilepsies. *Radiology, 225,* 880–887.

Morrow, L. A., Ryan, C. M., Hodgson, M. J., & Robin, N. (1990). Risk factors associated with persistence of neuropsychological deficits in persons with organic solvents exposure. *Journal of Nervous and Mental Disease, 179,* 540–545.

Morrow, L. A., Stein, L., Bagovich, G. R., Condray, R., & Scott, A. (2001). Neuropsychological assessment, depression, and past exposure to organic solvents. *Applied Neuropsychology, 8,* 65–73.

Mosher, D. L., & Smith, J. P. (1965). The usefulness of two scoring systems for the Bender gestalt test for identifying brain damage. *Journal of Consulting Psychology, 29,* 530–541.

Mueller, J., Kiernan, R. J., & Langston, J. W. (1988). The mental status examination. In H. H. Goldman (Ed.), *Review of general psychiatry.* Norwalk, CT: Appleton & Lange.

Nakase-Thompson, R., Manning, E., Sherer, M., Yablon, S. A., Gontkovsky, S. L. T, & Vickery, C. (2005). Brief assessment of severe language impairments: Initial validation of the Mississippi aphasia screening instrument. *Brain Injury, 19*, 685–691.

Nasrallah, H. A., & Weinberger, R. (1986). *The neurology of schizophrenia.* New York: Elsevier.

Natelson, B. H., Haupt, E. J., Fleisher, E. J., & Grey, L. (1979). Temporal orientation and education: A direct relationship in normal people. *Archives of Neurology, 36*, 444–446.

Navia, B. A., Jordan, B. D., & Price, R. W. (1986). The AIDS dementia complex I: Clinical features. *Annals of Neurology, 44*, 65–69.

Nelson, H. E. (1982). *National Adult Reading Test (NART): Test manual.* Windsor, UK: NFER Nelson.

Newcombe, F. (1969). *Missile wounds of the brain.* New York: Oxford University Press.

Newsome, M. R., Steinberg, J. L., Scheibel, R. S., Chu, Z., Lu, H., Lin, X., et al. (2008). Effects of traumatic brain injury on working memory-related brain activation in adolescents. *Neuropsychology, 22*, 419–425.

Newsome, M. R., Scheibel, R. S., Seignourel, P. J., Steinberg, J. L., Troyanskaya, M., Li, X., et al. (2009). Effects of methylphenidate on working memory in traumatic brain injury: A preliminary fMRI investigation. *Brain Imaging and Behavior, 3*, 298–305.

The Northern Neurobehavioral Group. (1988). *Manual for the Neurobehavioral Cognitive Status Examination.* Fairfax, CA: Author.

O'Donoghue, J. L. (1985). *Neurotoxicity of industrial and commercial chemicals* (Vols. I–II). Boca Raton, FL: CRC Press.

Olson, W. H., Brumback, R. A., Gascon, G., & Christoferson, L. A. (1981). *Practical neurology for the primary care physician.* Springfield, IL: Charles C Thomas.

Osterrieth, P. A. (1944). La test de copie d'une figure complexes. *Archives de Psychologie, 30*, 206–356.

Ott, B. R., Festa, E. K., Amick, M. M., Grace, J., Davis, J. D., & Heindel, W. C. (2008). Computerized maze navigation and performance by drivers with dementia. *Journal of Geriatric Psychiatry and Neurology, 21*(1), 18–25.

Ott, B. R., Heindel, W. C., Whelihan, W. M., Caron, M. D., Piatt, A. L., & DiCarlo, M. A. (2003). Maze test performance and reported driving ability in early dementia. *Journal of Geriatric Psychiatry and Neurology, 16.* Retrieved September 11, 2009, from http://jgp.sagepub.com/cgi/content/abstract/16/3/151

Owen, A. M., Morris, R. G., Sahakian, B. J., Polkey, C. E., & Robbins, T. W. (1996). Double dissociations of memory and executive functions in working memory tasks following frontal lobe excisions, temporal lobe excisions or amygdalo-hippocampectomy in man. *Brain, 119*, 1597–1615.

Oxbury, J. M., & Duchowny, M. (2000). Diagnosis and classification. In J. M. Oxbury, C. E. Polkey, & M. Duchowny (Eds.), *Intractable focal epilepsy.* London: W. B. Saunders.

Pajeau, A. K., & Roman, G. (1992). HIV encephalopathy and dementia. *Psychiatric Clinics of North America, 15*, 455–466.

Pankratz, L. (1983). A new technique for the assessment and modification of feigned memory deficit. *Perceptual and Motor Skills, 57*, 367–372.

Pankratz, L., Fausti, S. A., & Peed, S. (1975). A forced-choice technique to evaluate deafness in the hysterical or malingering patient. *Journal of Consulting and Clinical Psychology, 43*, 421–422.

Parsons, M. (1983). *Color atlas of clinical neurology.* Chicago: Year Book Medical Publishers.

Parsons, O. A. (1975). Brain damage in alcoholics: Altered states of unconsciousness. In M. M. Gross (Ed.), *Alcohol intoxication and withdrawal* (pp. 569–584). New York: Plenum Press.

Pascal, G. R., & Suttell, B. J. (1951). *The Bender-Gestalt Test: Quantification and validity for adults.* New York: Grune & Stratton.

Pataraia, E., Baumgartner, C., Lindinger, G., & Deecke, L. (2002). Magnetoencephalography in presurgical epilepsy evaluation. *Neurosurgery Review, 25*, 141–159.

Paul, D., Franzen, M. D., Fremouw, W., & Cohen, S. (1992). Standardization and validation of two tests used to detect malingering. *International Journal of Clinical Neuropsychology, 14*, 1–9.

Peters, R., & Pinto, E. M. (2008). Predictive value of the clock drawing test. *Dementia and Geriatric Cognitive Disorders, 26*, 351–355.

Pimental, P., & Kingsbury, W. (1989). *Mini Inventory of Right Brain Injury (MIRBI).* Austin, TX: Pro-Ed Publishers.

Pimental, P., & Knight, J. A. (1991, October). *A cross validation study of the mini-inventory of right brain injury (MIRBI).* Paper presented at the annual meeting of the National Academy of Neuropsychology, Dallas, TX.

Pincus, J. H., & Tucker, G. J. (1985). *Behavioral neurology* (3rd ed.). New York: Oxford University Press.

Pollak, Y., Kahana-Vax, G., & Hoofien, D. (2008). Retrieval processes in adults with ADHD: A RAVLT study, *Developmental Neuropsychology, 33*, 62–73.

Porteus, S. D. (1965). *Porteus Maze Tests: Fifty years' application.* Oxford, UK: Pacific Books.

Purdue Research Foundation. (1948). *Examiner's manual for the Purdue pegboard.* Chicago: Science Research Associates.

Rabin, L. A., Barr, W. B., & Burton, L. A. (2005). Assessment practices of clinical neuropsychologists in the United States and Canada: A survey of INS, NAN, and APA division 40 members. *Archives of Clinical Neuropsychology, 20*, 33–65.

Randolph, C., Tierney, M. C., Mohr, E., & Chase, T. N. (1998). The Repeatable Battery for the Assessment of Neuropsychological Status (RBANS): Preliminary clinical validity. *Journal of Clinical and Experimental Neuropsychology, 20*, 310–319.

Raven, J. C. (1960). *Guide to the standard progressive matrices.* London: H. K. Lewis.

Redmond, R., & Wilson, R. (1990). Neurological manifestations of AIDS. *Journal of the American Optometric Association, 61*, 760–766.

Reitan, R. M. (n.d.). *Instructions and procedures for administering the neuropsychological test battery used at the neuropsychology laboratory.* Unpublished manuscript, Indiana University Medical Center.

Reitan, R. M. (1958). Validity of the trail making test as an indicator of organic brain damage. *Perceptual and Motor Skills, 8*, 271–276.

Reitan, R. M., & Davison, L. A. (1974). *Clinical neuropsychology: Current status and applications.* Washington, DC: Winston/Wiley.
Reitan, R. M., & Wolfson, D. (1985). *The Halstead-Reitan neuropsychological test battery: Theory and clinical interpretation.* Tucson, AZ: Neuropsychology Press.
Reitan, R. M., & Wolfson, D. (2009). The Halstead Reitan Neuropsychological Battery: Theoretical, methodological and validational bases (3rd ed.,pp. 3–24). In I. Grant & K. M. Adams (Eds.), *Neuropsychological assessment of neuropsychiatric and neuromedical disorders.* New York: Oxford University Press.
Rey, A. (1941). L'examen psychologique dans les cas d'encephalopathie traumatique. *Archives de Psychologie, 28,* 286–340.
Rey, A. (1964). *L'examen clinique en psychologie (English chapter summaries).* Paris: Presses Universitaires de France.
Reynolds, C. R., & Gutkin, T. B. (1979). Predicting the premorbid intellectual status of children using demographic data. *Clinical Neuropsychology, 1,* 36–38.
Roid, G. (2003). *The Stanford-Binet Intelligence Scale* (5th ed.). Rolling Meadows, IL: Riverside Publishing.
Rosselli, M., & Ardila, A. (1991). Effects of age, education, and gender on the Rey-Osterreith complex figure. *Clinical Neuropsychologist, 5,* 370–376.
Roselli, M., Tartaglione, B., Federico, F., Lepore, V., Defazio, G., & Livrea, P. (2009). Rate of MMSE score change in Alzheimer's disease: Influence of education and vascular risk factors. *Clinical Neurology and Neurosurgery, 111,* 327–330.
Ruocco, A. C., Swirsky-Sacchetti, T., Chute, D. L., Mandel, S., Platek, S. M., & Zillmer, E. A. (2008). Distinguishing between neuropsychological malingering and exaggerated psychiatric symptoms in a neuropsychological setting. *Clinical Neuropsychologist, 22,* 547–564.
Russell, E. W. (1975). A multiple scoring method for the assessment of complex memory functions. *Journal of Consulting and Clinical Psychology, 43,* 800–809.
Russell, E. W., Neuringer, C., & Goldstein, G. (1970). *Assessment of brain damage: A neuropsychological key approach.* New York: John Wiley Interscience.
Sacktor, N. (2002). The epidemiology of human immunodeficiency virus associated neurological disease in the era of highly active antiretroviral therapy. *Journal of Neurovirology, 8,* 115–121.
Salter, K., Jutai, J., Foley, N., Hellings, C., & Teasell, R. (2006). Identification of aphasia post stroke: A review of screening assessment tools. *Brain Injury, 20*(6), 559–568.
Salthouse, T. A., & Fristoe, N. M. (1995). Process analysis of adult age effects on a computer-administered trail making test. *Georgia Institute of Technology, 9,* 518–528.
Schamhorst, S. (1992). AIDS dementia complex in the elderly: Diagnosis and management. *Nurse Practitioner, 17,* 41–43.
Schatz, P., & Browndyke, J. (2002). Applications of computer-based neuropsychological assessment. *Journal of Head Trauma Rehabilitation, 17*(5), 395–410.
Schmidt, K. S., Lieto, J. M., Kiryankova, E., & Salvucci, A. (2006). Construct and concurrent validity of the dementia rating scale-2 alternate form. *Journal of Clinical and Experimental Neuropsychology, 28,* 646–654.
Schmidt, K. S., Mattis, P. J., Adams, J., & Nestor, P. (2005). Test-retest reliability of the Dementia Rating Scale-2: Alternate Form. *Dementia and Geriatric Cognitive Disorders, 20*(1), 42–44.

Schmidt, M. (1996). *Rey Auditory and Verbal Learning Test: A handbook*. Los Angeles, CA: Western Psychological Services.

Schoenberg, M. R., Dawson, K. A., Duff, K., Patton, D., Scott, J. G., & Adams, R. L. (2006). Test performance and classification statistics for the Rey auditory verbal learning test in selected clinical samples. *Archives of Clinical Neuropsychology, 21*, 693–703.

Schrimsher, G. W., O'Bryant, S. E., Parker, J. D., & Burke, R. S. (2005). The relation between ethnicity and Cognistat performance in males seeking substance use disorder treatment. *Journal of Clinical and Experimental Neuropsychology, 27*, 873–885.

Schwamm, L. H., van Dyke, C., Kiernan, R. J., Merrin, E. L., & Mueller, J. (1987). The Neurobehavioral Cognitive Status Examination: Comparison with the Cognitive Capacity Screening Examination and the Mini-Mental State Examination in a neurosurgical population. *Annals of Internal Medicine, 107*, 486–491.

Sherman, D. S., Boone, K. B., Lu, P., & Razani, J. (2002). Re-examination of a Rey auditory verbal learning test/Rey complex figure discriminant function to detect suspect effort. *Clinical Neuropsychologist, 16*(3), 242–250.

Sherrill, R. E. (1985). Comparison of three short forms of the category test. *Journal of Clinical and Experimental Neuropsychology, 7*, 231–238.

Sherrill, R. E. (1987). Options for shortening Halstead's category test for adults. *Archives of Clinical Neuropsychology, 2*, 343–352.

Sheslow, D. V., & Adams, W. V. (2003). *Wide range assessment of memory and learning* (2nd ed.). Wilmington, DE: Wide Range.

Sivan, A. B. (1991). *Benton visual retention test* (5th ed.). San Antonio, TX: Psychological Corporation.

Smith, R. L., Goode, K. T., La Marche, J. A., & Boll, T. J. (1995). Selective reminding test short form administration: A comparison of two through twelve trials. *Psychological Assessment, 7*(2), 177–182.

Snow, R. B., Zimmerman, R. D., Gandy, S. E., & Deck, M. D. F. (1986). Comparison of magnetic resonance imaging and computed tomography in the evaluation of head injury. *Neurosurgery, 18*, 45–52.

Spencer, T. J., Biederman, J., Wilens, T. E., & Faraone, S. V. (2002). Overview and neurobiology of attention-deficit hyperactivity disorder. *Journal of Clinical Psychiatry, 63*, 3–9.

Spreen, O., & Benton, A. L. (1977). *Neurosurgery center comprehensive examination for aphasia*. Victoria, BC, Canada: University of Victoria Neuropsychology Laboratory.

Spreen, O., & Risser, A. H. (2003). *Assessment of aphasia*. New York: Oxford University Press.

Spreen, O., Sherman, E. M. S., & Strauss, E. (2006). *A compendium of neuropsychological tests: Administration, norms, and commentary* (2nd ed.). New York: Oxford University Press.

Stankoff, B., Tourbah, A., Suarez, S., Turrell, E., Stienvart, J. L., Payan, C., et al. (2001). Clinical and spectroscopic improvement in HIV-associated cognitive impairment. *Neurology, 56*, 112–115.

Starrat, C., Fields, R. B., & Cisewski, D. (1992, November). *An update on the validity of the MMSE*. Paper presented at the annual meeting of the National Academy of Neuropsychology, Pittsburgh, PA.

Stebbins, G. T., Wilson, R. S., Gilley, D. W., Bernard, B. A., & Fox, J. H. (1990). Use of the national adult reading test to estimate premorbid IQ in dementia. *Clinical Neuropsychologist, 4*, 18–24.

Steck, P. H. (2005). A revision of A. L. Benton's visual retention test in two parallel forms. *Archives of Clinical Neuropsychology, 20*, 409–416.

Stephan, B. C., & Brayne, C. (2008). Vascular factors and prevention of dementia. *International Review of Psychiatry, 20*, 344–356.

Stern, R. A., & White, T. (2003). *Neuropsychological assessment battery*. Lutz, FL: Psychological Assessment Battery.

Strakowski, S. M., DelBello, M. P., & Adler, C. M. (2005). The functional neuroanatomy of bipolar disorder. *Molecular Psychiatry, 10*, 105–116.

Strakowski, S. M., McElroy, S. L., Keck, P. E., Jr., & West, S. A. (1996). Racial influence on diagnosis in psychotic mania. *Journal of Affective Disorders, 39*, 157–162.

Strauss, E., Sherman, E. S., & Spreen, O. (2006). *A compendium of neuropsychological tests: Administration, norms, and commentary* (3rd ed.). New York: Oxford University Press.

Street, R. F. (1931). *A Gestalt Completion Test. Contributions to education, No. 481*. New York: Bureau of Publications, Teachers College, Columbia University.

Stroop, J. R. (1935). The basis of Ligon's theory. *American Journal of Psychology, 47*, 499–504.

Strub, R. L., & Black, F. W. (1977). *The mental status examination in neurology*. Philadelphia: F. A. Davis.

Strub, R. L., & Black, F. W. (1988). *Organic brain syndromes: An introduction to neurobehavioral disorders* (2nd ed.). Philadelphia: F. A. Davis.

Strub, R. L., & Black, F. W. (1993). *The mental status exam in neurology* (3rd ed.). Philadelphia: F. A. Davis.

Sturges, J. W. (1998). Practical use of technology in professional practice. *Professional Psychology Research and Practice, 29*, 183–188.

Sullivan, K., Deffenti, C., & Keane, B. (2002). Malingering on the RAVLT part II. Detection strategies. *Archives of Clinical Neuropsychology, 17*, 223–233.

Sunderland, T., Hill, J. L., Mellow, A. M., Lawlor, B. A., Gundersheimer, J., Newhouse, P. A., et al. (1989). Clock drawing in Alzheimer's disease: A novel measure of dementia severity. *Journal of the American Geriatrics Society, 37*, 725–729.

Swanson, J. M., Flodman, P., Kennedy, J., Spence, M. A., Moyzis, R., Schuck, S., et al. (2000). Dopamine genes and ADHD. *Neuroscience Biobehavioral Review, 24*, 21–25.

Taylor, R. (1982). *Mind or body: Distinguishing psychological from organic disorders*. New York: McGraw-Hill.

Teasdale, G., & Jennett, B. (1974). Assessment of coma and impaired consciousness. *Lancet, 2*(7872), 81–83.

Thurstone, L. L. (1938). *Primary mental abilities*. Chicago: University of Chicago Press.

Thurstone, L. L., & Thurstone, T. G. (1962). *Primary mental abilities* (rev. ed.). Chicago: Science Research Associates.

Tien, A. Y., Spevack, T. V., Jones, D. W., Pearlson, G. D., Schlaepfer, T. E., & Strauss, M. E. (1996). Computerized Wisconsin card sorting test: Comparison with manual administration. *Kaohsiung Journal of Medical Science, 12*, 479–485.

Tolor, A., & Schulberg, H. (1963). *An evaluation of the Bender-Gestalt*. Springfield, IL: Charles C Thomas.
Tombaugh, T. N. (1996). *The Test of Memory Malingering (TOMM)*. Toronto, Canada: Multi-Health Systems.
Tombaugh, T. N., & Hubley, A. M. (1997). The 60-item Boston Naming Test: Norms for cognitively intact adults aged 25–88 years. *Journal of Clinical and Experimental Neuropsychology, 14,* 167–177.
Tow, P. M. (1955). *Personality changes following frontal leucotomy*. New York: Oxford University Press.
Trauner, D. A. (1982). Seizure disorder. In W. G. Wiederholt (Ed.), *Neurology for non-neurologists* (pp. 283–297). New York: Academic Press.
Tymchuk, A. J. (1974). Comparison of the Bender error and time scores from groups of epileptic, retarded, and behavior problem children. *Perceptual and Motor Skills, 38,* 71–79.
Tzavaras, A., Hecaen, H., & Le Bras, H. (1970). Le probleme de la specificite du deficit de la reconnaissance du visage humain lors des lesions hemispheriques unilaterales. *Neuropsychologia, 8,* 403–416.
Uddo, M., Vasterling, J., Brailey, K., & Sutker, P. (1993). Memory and attention in combat-related post-traumatic stress disorder. *Journal of Psychopathology and Behavioural Assessment, 15,* 43–52.
Vickery, C. D., Berry, D. T. R., Inman, T. H., Harris, M. J., & Orey, S. A. (2001). Detection of inadequate effort on neuropsychological testing: A meta-analytic review of selected procedures. *Archives of Clinical Neuropsychology, 16,* 45–73.
Volbrecht, M. E., Meyers, J. E., & Kaster-Bundgaard, J. (2000). Neuropsychological outcome of head injury using a short battery. *Archives of Clinical Neuropsychology, 15,* 251–264.
Walsh, M. C., Groisser, D., & Pennington, B. F. (1988). *A normative-developmental study of performance on measures hypothesized to tap prefrontal functions*. Paper presented to the International Neuropsychological Society, New Orleans, LA.
Wang, P. L. (1984). *Manual for the modified Vygotsky concept formation test*. Chicago: Stoelting.
Wang, P. L. (1990). Assessment of cognitive competency. In D. E. Tupper & K. D. Cicerone (Eds.), *The neuropsychology of everyday life: Assessment and basic competencies*. Boston: Kluwer Academic Publishers.
Wang, P. L., & Ennis, K. E. (1986). Competency assessment in clinical populations: An introduction to the cognitive competency test. In B. Uzzell & Y. Gross (Eds.), *Clinical neuropsychology of intervention*. Boston: Martinus Nijhoff.
Wang, P. L., Ennis, K., & Copeland, S. (1987). *Cognitive competency test*. Toronto, ON, Canada: Mount Sinai Hospital, Psychology Department.
Warrington, E. K., & James, M. (1967). Disorders of visual perception in patients with localized cerebral lesions. *Neuropsychologia, 5,* 253–266.
Warrington, E. K., & Rabin, P. (1970). Perceptual matching in patients with cerebral lesions. *Neuropsychology, 8,* 475–487.
Watson, C. G. (1968). The separation of neuropsychiatric hospital organics from schizophrenics with three visual motor screening tests. *Journal of Clinical Psychology, 24,* 412–414.

Wechsler, D. (1987). *Wechsler Memory Scale–Revised manual.* San Antonio, TX: Psychological Corporation.
Wechsler, D. (2009). *Wechsler Memory Scale-IV Manual.* San Antonio, TX: Psychological Corporation.
Wechsler, D. A. (1945). A standardized memory scale for clinical use. *Journal of Psychology, 19,* 87–95.
Wechsler, D. A. (1981). *Manual for the Wechsler Adult Intelligence Scale–Revised.* New York: Psychological Corporation.
Wechsler, D. A. (1997). *Manual for the Wechsler Adult Intelligence Scale–III.* San Antonio, TX: Psychological Corporation.
Wechsler, D. A. (2002). *Wechsler Individual Achievement Test* (2nd ed.). San Antonio, TX: The Psychological Corporation.
Wechsler, D. A. (2008). *The Wechsler Adult Intelligence Scale* (4th ed.). San Antonio, TX: The Psychological Corporation.
Wedding, D. (1986). Neurological disorders. In D. Wedding, A. M. Horton, Jr., & J. Webster (Eds.), *The neuropsychology handbook: Behavioral and clinical perspectives* (pp. 59–79). New York: Springer Publishing Company.
Weigl, E. (1941). On the psychology of so-called processes of abstraction. *Journal of Abnormal and Social Psychology, 36,* 3–33.
Weinstein, S. (1964). Deficits concomitant with aphasia or lesions of either cerebral hemisphere. *Cortex, 1,* 151–169.
Wells, C. E., & Duncan, G. W. (1980). *Neurology for psychiatrists.* Philadelphia: F. A. Davis.
Wiederholt, W. C. (1982). Cerebrovascular disease. In W. C. Wiederholt (Ed.), *Neurology for non-neurologists* (pp. 179–189). New York: Academic Press.
Wiederholt, W. C. (1982). Dementias. In W. C. Wiederholt (Ed.), *Neurology for non-neurologists* (pp. 191–203). New York: Academic Press.
Wilkinson, G. S., & Robertson, G. J. (2006). *WRAT-4: The Wide Range Achievement Test administration manual* (4th ed.). Wilmington, DE: Wide Range.
Wilson, B., Cockburn, J., & Baddeley, A. (1985). *The Rivermead behavioural memory test. Reading.* Fareham, UK: Thames Valley Test Company.
Wilson, R. S., Schneider, J. A., Arnold, S. E., Tang, Y., Boyle, P. A., & Bennett, D. A. (2007). Olfactory identification and incidence of mild cognitive impairment in older age. *Archives of General Psychiatry, 64,* 802–808.
Wolf, J. K. (1980). *Practical clinical neurology.* Garden City, NY: Medical Examination Publishing.
Wolf-Klein, G. P., Silverstone, F. A., Levy, A. P., & Brod, M. S. (1989). Screening for Alzheimer's disease by clock drawing. *Journal of the American Psychiatric Association, 37,* 730–734.
Woodcock, R. W. (1973). *Woodcock Reading Mastery Tests.* Circle Pines, MN: American Guidance Service.
Wysocki, J. J., & Sweet, J. J. (1985). Identification of brain-damaged, schizophrenic, and normal medical patients using a brief neuropsychological screening battery. *International Journal of Clinical Neuropsychology, 7,* 40–44.
Yazdanfar, D. J. (1990). Assessing the mental status of the cognitively impaired elderly. *Journal of Gerontological Nursing, 16,* 32–36.

Yehuda, R., Keefe, R., Harvey, P., Levengood, R., Gerber, D., Geni, J., et al. (1995). Learning and memory in combat veterans with posttraumatic stress disorder. *American Journal of Psychiatry, 152,* 137–139.

York Haaland, K., Vranes, L. F., Goodwin, J. S., & Garry, J. P. (1987). Wisconsin card sorting test performance in a healthy elderly population. *Journal of Gerontology, 42,* 345–346.

Zangwill, O. L. (1966). Psychological deficits associated with frontal lobe lesions. *International Journal of Neurology, 5,* 395–402.

Index

A
Abnormal word usage, 57–58
Abstract reasoning, 97–98
Abstract Words Test, 156–157
Acquired immunodeficiency syndrome, 69
Acromegaly, 35
ADHD. *See* Attention-deficit/hyperactivity disorders
Affective disorders, 35–37
  acromegaly, 35
  anemia, 35
  Controlled Word Association Test, 36
  Cushing's disease, 35
  dementia, depression, differential diagnosis, 35–36
  Minnesota Multiphasic Personality Inventory, 37
  multiple sclerosis, 35
  parathyroid disease, 35
  Parkinson's disease, 36
  pseudodementia, 36
  systemic lupus erythematosus, 35
  thyroid disease, 35
  ulcerative colitis, 35
Agraphia, 10
AIDS. *See* Acquired immunodeficiency syndrome
AIDS-related dementia. *See* Human immunodeficiency virus dementia
Alcohol, 13
Alcoholism, 3, 39–40
  Korsakoff's psychosis, 39–40
  Wernicke-Korsakoff syndrome, 40
Alzheimer's disease, 11–14
Anemia, 35
Anosognosia, 7
Anoxia, schizophrenia-like episodes, 34
Anterior cerebral artery infarcts, 7
Anxiety, 20, 37–38. *See also* Wilson's disease
  dysregulation of hypothalamic-pituitary-adrenal axis, 38
  generalized anxiety disorder, 38
  obsessive-compulsive disorder, 38
  posttraumatic stress disorder, 38
Aphasia Screening Test, 126
Apolipoprotein E, 14
Apoplexy, 5–6
Army individual test. *See* Trail Making Test
Arsenic, lead, mercury, thallium, 13
Arteriovenous malformation, 12
AST. *See* Aphasia Screening Test
Astrocytomas, 5
Ataxia, 10
Atherosclerosis, 6
Athetosis, 18
Attention, 85–88
  homonomous hemianopsia, 87
  random letters procedure, 85–86
  vigilance, 85
  Wechsler Adult Intelligence Scale–Revised, 85
Attention-deficit/hyperactivity disorders, 38–39
Auditory functions, 117–118
Autoimmune diseases, schizophrenia-like episodes, 34
Average evoked potentials, 49

B
Barona IQ estimate equations, 164
Behavior patterns, 72
Bender Visual-Motor Gestalt Test, 108–109, 162
Benton Visual Retention Test, 109–111
Bilateral simultaneous stimulation, 4
Binswanger's disease, 12
Block design test, 112
Boston Naming Test, 132
Bowel function, 3
Brain electrical activity mapping, 49

Brain lacerations, 24
Brain tumors, 2–5
  alcoholism, 3
  astrocytomas, 5
  benign tumors, 4
  bilateral simultaneous stimulation, 4
  bowel function, 3
  brainstem, tumors arising in, 5
  cerebellum, tumors arising in, 5
  cerebral tumors, 2
  classifying, 4
  ependymomas, 5
  extrinsic tumors, 4
  glioblastoma multiforme, 5
  gliomas, 5
  head trauma, 3
  headaches, 2
  intracranial pressure, 3
  intrinsic tumors, 4
  limbic system tumors, 2
  malignant tumors, 4
  medulloblastomas, 5
  neoplastic disease clinical presentation, 2–4
  oligodendrogliomas, 5
  papilledema, 3
  projectile vomiting, 2
  seizures, 2
  slow-growing tumors, 3
Brainstem, tumors arising in, 5
Brief Visuospatial Memory Test–Revised, 147
Buschke Selective Reminding Test, record form, 146
BVRT. *See* Benton Visual Retention Test

C
California Verbal Learning Test, 189
Cambridge Neuropsychological Test Automated Batteries, 197
CANTAB. *See* Cambridge Neuropsychological Test Automated Batteries
Carbon monoxide, 13
Carotid artery occlusive disease, 12
Catatonic schizophrenia, 33
Categorical fluency, 133–134
Category Test, 161, 195

Cerebellum, tumors arising in, 5
Cerebral angiography, 53
Cerebral anoxia, schizophrenia-like episodes, 34
Cerebral embolism, 12
Cerebral tumors, 2
Cerebrospinal fluid, 9
Cerebrovascular accidents, 5–7
Changes in sexual behavior, 69
Charcot's triad, 19
Circle of Willis, 6
Classification of epilepsy, 26–27
Clinical magnetoencephalography, 50
Clock drawing, 113–114
Color Form Sorting Test, 158–159
Color perception, 105–106
Color Sorting Test, 157–158
Coma, 79
Commercially available computerized assessments, 196–197
Complement receptor 1, 14
Computed tomography, 41, 50
Computerized assessments, 193–198
  Cambridge Neuropsychological Test Automated Batteries, 197
  Category Test from Halstead-Reitan Neuropsychological Test Battery, 195
  commercially available computerized assessments, 196–197
  computer tests, 193–195
  Conner's Continuous Performance Task, 196–197
  with functional magnetic resonance imaging, 194–195
  Immediate Postconcussion Assessment and Cognitive Testing, 197
  Iowa Gambling Task, 197
  Peabody Picture Vocabulary Test, 196
  Raven's Progressive Matrices, 196
  traditional paper-and-pencil tests, computerized versions, 195–196
  Wechsler Adult Intelligence Scale, 193
  Wisconsin Card Sorting Test, 195
Concept formation, tests of, 155–161
  Abstract Words Test, 156–157
  Proverbs Test, 156
  sorting tests, 157–161

Concussions, 23
Conner's Continuous Performance Task, 196–197
Consciousness level, 78–80
  alert, 79
  coma, 79
  lethargy, 79
  semicoma, 79
  stupor, 79
Construction tests, 112
Constructional abilities, 94–96
Contralateral sensory loss, 7
Controlled Oral Word Association Test, 58
Controlled Word Association Test, 36, 133
Contusions, 23–24
CPT-II. *See* Conner's Continuous Performance Task
CR1. *See* Complement receptor 1
Cranial nerves, 44–46
Creutzfeldt-Jacob disease, 13
CSF. *See* Cerebrospinal fluid
CT. *See* Computed tomography
Current litigation, 73
Current living situation, 73
Cushing's disease, 12, 35
CVAs. *See* Cerebrovascular accidents
CVLT. *See* California Verbal Learning Test

D
Degenerative disease
  of CNS, 12
  schizophrenia-like episodes, 34
Dementia, 7, 11–22
  AIDS-related, 20–22
  Alzheimer's disease, 11–14
  Binswanger's disease, 12
  cerebral embolism, 12
  Charcot's triad, 19
  Creutzfeldt-Jacob disease, 13
  Cushing's disease, 12
  depression, differential diagnosis, 35–36
  dialysis encephalopathy, 12
  echolalia, 17
  electrolyte disturbances, 12
  encephalitis, 13
  endocrine disease, 12
  epilepsy, 13
  Hirano bodies, 14
  human immunodeficiency virus dementia, 20–22
  Huntington's chorea, 12, 18–19
  hypercalcemia, 12
  hyperthyroidism, 12
  hypocalcemia, 12
  hypopituitarism, 12
  hypothyroidism, 12
  intracranial space-occupying lesions, 13
  Kayser-Fleischer ring, 20
  Kluver-Bucy syndrome, 17
  kuru, 13
  metabolic disease, 12
  multiple sclerosis, 13, 19
  muscular dystrophy, 13
  neurofibrillary tangles, 14
  normal pressure hydrocephalus, 13
  nutritional disease, 12
  organic solvents, 13
  palmomental reflex, 15–16
  Parkinson's disease, 12, 17–18
  penicillamine, 20
  Pick's disease, 12, 16
  progressive supranuclear palsy, 12
  renal failure, 12
  reversible causes, 14
  rooting reflex, 15
  snout reflex, 15
  subarachnoid hemorrhage, 12
  syphilis, 13
  toxins, 13
  vascular disorder, 12
  vitamin deficiency, 12
  Wechsler Adult Intelligence Scale–Revised, 15
  Wechsler Memory Scale–Revised, 16
  Wernicke-Korsakoff syndrome, 12
  Wilson's disease, 12, 19–20
Depression, 20. *See also* Wilson's disease
Design recognition, 107–108
Diabetes, 8
Dialysis encephalopathy, 12
Digit span, 141–142

Discrimination test, 118–120
Disorganized schizophrenia, 33
Drug abuse, 71–72
Dysartbria, 58
Dysarthria, 10
Dysfluency, 58
Dysregulation of hypothalamic-pituitary-adrenal axis, 38

E
Echolalia, 17
Effort, 185–191
  California Verbal Learning Test, 189
  Forced-Choice Test of Nonverbal Ability, 188–189
  Reliable Digit Span, 190
  Rey Auditory-Verbal Learning Test, 189–190
  Rey Memory for 15 Items Test, 187–188
  Symptom Validity Testing, 188
  Test of Memory Malingering, 190
  Wechsler Adult Intelligence Scale, Third Edition, 190
Electroencephalography, 41, 48–49
Electrolyte disturbances, 12
Electromyograph, 41
Embolus, 8
EMG. *See* Electromyograph
Emotional stress, 26
Encephalitis, 13
  schizophrenia-like episodes, 34
Endocrine disease, 12
Endogenous depression, 10
Environmental stimuli, 26
Ependymomas, 5
Epilepsy, 13, 25–29
Evoked potentials, 49
Executive functioning, 154
Expressive aphasia, 7
Extrinsic tumors, 4

F
Face recognition, 107
Family history, 63–64
FAST. *See* Frenchay Aphasia Screening Test
Fever, 26
Figure recognition, 107–108

Finger Tapping Test, 121–122
fMRI. *See* Functional magnetic resonance imaging
Folate deficiency, 12
Forced-Choice Test of Nonverbal Ability, 188–189
Forensic information, 72
Frenchay Aphasia Screening Test, 129
Functional magnetic resonance imaging, 52–53, 194–195

G
GAD. *see* Generalized anxiety disorder
Galveston Orientation and Amnesia Test, 83
Generalized anxiety disorder, 38
Generalized seizures, 28–29
Generalized tonic-clonic seizures, 29
Glasgow Coma Scale, 24, 80–81
Glioblastoma multiforme, 5
Gliomas, 5
GOAT. *See* Galveston Orientation and Amnesia Test
Grand mal seizures, 29
Grip strength, 122

H
Hallucinations, 28
Halstead-Reitan Battery, 9
Halstead-Reitan Neuropsychological Test Battery, 126, 195
Head trauma, 3, 13, 22–25
  brain lacerations, 24
  concussions, 23
  contusions, 23–24
  Glasgow Coma Scale, 24
  open-head injuries, 23–24
  postconcussion syndrome, 23
  posttraumatic amnesia, 24–25
  repeated concussions, 23
Headaches, 2
Heavy metals, 13
Hemianopsia, 7, 87
Hemorrhage, 7
Hepatic failure, 12
Hepatolenticular degeneration, 19–20
Higher cognitive functions, 96–98, 153–165
  abstract reasoning, 97–98

concept formation, tests of, 155–161
executive functioning, 154
general information, 97
organizational/planning abilities, 161–164
proverb interpretation, 97–98
similarities, 97
Wisconsin Card Sorting Test, 153
Hirano bodies, 14
History, 43
Hopkins Verbal Learning Test–Revised, 143–144
Hormonal changes, 26
Human immunodeficiency virus dementia, 20–22
Human social interaction, 72
Huntington's chorea, 12, 18–19
Hyperactivity, 38–39
Hypercalcemia, 12
Hypertension, 6, 8
Hyperthyroidism, 12
Hyperventilation, 26
Hypocalcemia, 12
Hypopituitarism, 12
Hypothyroidism, 12

I
IGT. See Iowa Gambling Task
Immediate Postconcussion Assessment and Cognitive Testing, 197
ImPACT. See Immediate Postconcussion Assessment and Cognitive Testing
Impairment Index, 9
Infarcts, 7–8
Infections, 13
International Classification of Epileptic Seizures, 26
Intracranial pressure, 3
Intracranial space-occupying lesions, 13
Intrinsic tumors, 4
Iowa Gambling Task, 197
Ischemia, 8

K
Kayser-Fleischer ring, 20
Kluver-Bucy syndrome, 17
Kuru, 13

L
Language, 88–91
Language abnormalities, 57–58
abnormal word usage, 57–58
Controlled Oral Word Association Test, 58
dysartbria, 58
dysfluency, 58
mispronunciation, 57–58
Peabody Picture Vocabulary Test–Revised, 58
Lead, 13
Lethargy, 79
Limbic system tumors, 2
Litigation, 73
Lumbar puncture, 53–54

M
Magnetic resonance imaging, 41, 52
Magnetoencephalography, 50
Malignant tumors, 4
Mania, 20. See also Wilson's disease
Manual motor functioning, 121–123
    Finger Tapping Test, 121–122
    grip strength, 122
    Purdue Pegboard Test, 122–123
Mattis Dementia Rating Scale, 150
Medical history, 70–73
    abuse of drugs, 71–72
    behavior patterns, 72
    drug abuse, 71–72
    forensic information, 72
    human social interaction, 72
    premorbid personality, 72
    psychiatric history, 71
    suicide attempts, 71
    surgery, 70
Medulloblastomas, 5
Memory, 91–94
    short-term memory, 92
    spatial memory, 91
    verbal memory, 91
    visual memory, 91, 93
    visual-spatial memory, 93
    Wechsler Memory Scale, 91
Memory functions screening, 139–151
    Buschke Selective Reminding Test, record form, 146
    memory test batteries, 148–150
    verbal memory, learning problems, 140–145

visual memory functioning, 145–148
Wechsler Adult Intelligence Scale–Fourth Edition, 139
Memory test batteries, 148–150
  Mattis Dementia Rating Scale, 150
  Rivermead Behavioral Memory Test, 150
  Wechsler Memory Scale–IV, 148–149
  Wide Range Assessment of Memory and Learning–Second Edition, 149–150
Meningitis, 13
Mental status examination, 75–102
  applications, 98–99
  attention, 85–88
  brief evaluations, 99–101
  complex functions, 98
  constructional abilities, 94–96
  Glasgow Coma Scale, 80–81
  higher cognitive functions, 96–98
  language, 88–91
  level of consciousness, 78–80
  memory, 91–94
  Mini-Mental State Exam, 100–101
  orientation, 83–85
  Rancho Los Amigos Scale, 81–83
Mercury, 13
Metabolic disease, 12
Micrographia, 17
Mini-Mental State Exam, 100–101
Minnesota Multiphasic Personality Inventory, 37
Mispronunciation, 57–58
MMPI-II. *See* Minnesota Multiphasic Personality Inventory
MMSE. *See* Mini-Mental State Exam
Motivation, 185–191
  California Verbal Learning Test, 189
  Forced-Choice Test of Nonverbal Ability, 188–189
  Reliable Digit Span, 190
  Rey Auditory-Verbal Learning Test, 189–190
  Rey Memory for 15 Items Test, 187–188
  Symptom Validity Testing, 188
  Test of Memory Malingering, 190
  Wechsler Adult Intelligence Scale, Third Edition, 190
Motor, perceptual function screening, 103–123
  auditory functions, 117–118
  manual motor functioning, 121–123
  spatial abilities, complex visual functions-tests, 108–117
  tactile functions, 118–121
  visual functions, 104–106
  visual recognition, 106–108
Motor abnormalities, 58–60
  abnormalities of symmetry, 59
Movement, 43–44
MRI. *See* Magnetic resonance imaging
MS. *See* Multiple sclerosis
MSE. *See* Mental status examination
Multifocal leukoencephalopathy, 13
Multi-infarct dementia, 12
Multiple sclerosis, 13, 19, 35
Muscular dystrophy, 13

N
Neoplasms, schizophrenia-like episodes, 34
Neoplastic disease clinical presentation, 2–4
Neurofibrillary tangles, 14
Neurological assessment, 41–54
  arousal, 43
  average evoked potentials, 49
  brain electrical activity mapping, 49
  cerebral angiography, 53
  clinical magnetoencephalography, 50
  computed tomography, 41
  cranial nerves, 44–46
  CT scan, 50
  electroencephalography, 41, 48–49
  electromyograph, 41
  functional magnetic resonance imaging, 52–53
  history, 43
  lumbar puncture, 53–54
  magnetic resonance imaging, 41, 52
  movement, 43–44
  positron emission tomography scans, 51
  posture, 43–44
  reflexes, 47–48
  regional cerebral blood flow, 50–51

sensation, tests of, 46
single-photon emission computerized tomography, 41, 51
skull radiographs, 50
strength, tests of, 47–48
tone, tests of, 47–48
Neurological disorders, 1–30
  brain tumors, 2–5
  dementias, 11–22
  head trauma, 22–25
  seizure disorders, 25–29
  vascular disorders, 5–11
  Wilson's disease, suicide rate, 20
Neuropsychological history, 55–73
  acquired immunodeficiency syndrome, 69
  appearance of subject, 56–57
  changes in sexual behavior, 69
  current complaints, 61–63
  current litigation, 73
  current living situation, 73
  current situation, 73
  early history, 65–66
  family history, 63–64
  identification of patient, 61
  language abnormalities, 57–58
  medical history, 70–73
  motor abnormalities, 58–60
  obtaining history, 60–73
  occupational history, 66–68
  prenatal history, 64–65
  sexual history, 68–69
  Wechsler Adult Intelligence Scale–IV, 55
Neuropsychological screening, 167–184
  Barry Rehabilitation Inpatient Screening of Cognition, 174–175
  Boston Process approach, 167
  Cognitive Competency Test, 178–180
  Halstead-Reitan, 167
  Kaufman Short Neuropsychological Assessment Procedure, 181–184
  Luria-Nebraska Batteries, 167
  Middlesex Elderly Assessment of Mental State, 181
  Mini-Inventory of Right-Brain Injury, 180–181
  Neurobehavioral Cognitive Status Examination, 176–178

Neuropsychological Assessment Battery, 176
  Repeatable Battery for Assessment of Neuropsychological Status, 175–176
Niacin deficiency, 12
Normal pressure hydrocephalus, 13
Nutritional disease, 12

O
Object Sorting Test, 159
Obsessive-compulsive disorder, 38
Obstructive strokes, 8
Occlusions, 7
Occupational history, 66–68
OCD. *See* Obsessive-compulsive disorder
Oligodendrogliomas, 5
Open-head injuries, 23–24
Optic disc swelling. *See* Papilledema
Organic solvents, 13
Organizational/planning abilities, 161–164
  Barona IQ estimate equations, 164
  Bender Visual-Motor Gestalt designs, 162
  Porteus Maze test, 162
  premorbid functioning estimation, 162–164
Orientation, 83–85
  Galveston Orientation and Amnesia Test, 83

P
Palmomental reflex, 15–16
Papilledema, 3
Parathyroid disease, 35
Paranoid schizophrenia, 33
Paranoid thinking, 20. *See also* Wilson's disease
Parkinson's disease, 12, 17–18, 36
Partial seizures, 26–27
Peabody Picture Vocabulary Test, 58, 106, 196
Penicillamine, 20
Perceptual, motor functions screening, 103–123
  auditory functions, 117–118
  manual motor functioning, 121–123
  spatial abilities, complex visual functions-tests, 108–117

tactile functions, 118–121
visual functions, 104–106
visual recognition, 106–108
Pick's disease, 12, 16
Porteus Maze test, 162
Positron emission tomography scans, 51
Postconcussion syndrome, 23
Posterior cerebral artery infarcts, 7
Posttraumatic amnesia, 24–25
  severity of injury, relationship, 25
Posttraumatic stress disorder, 38
Posture, 43–44
PPVT. *See* Peabody Picture Vocabulary Test
Premorbid functioning estimation, 162–164
Premorbid personality, 72
Prenatal history, 64–65
Progressive supranuclear palsy, 12
Projectile vomiting, 2
Proverb interpretation, 97–98
Proverbs Test, 156
Pseudodementia, 36
Psychiatric disorders, 31–40
  affective disorders, 35–37
  alcoholism, 39–40
  anxiety disorders, 37–38
  attention-deficit/hyperactivity disorders, 38–39
  schizophrenia, 31–35
Psychiatric history, 71
Psychiatric symptoms of Wilson's disease, 20
PTSD. *See* Posttraumatic stress disorder
Purdue Pegboard Test, 122–123

R
Rancho Los Amigos Scale, 81–83
Random letters procedure, 85–86
Raven's Progressive Matrices, 112–113, 196
RAVLT. *See* Rey Auditory-Verbal Learning Test
Reading fluency, 134–137
  academic skills, 136–137
  Stroop Test, 134–136
Reflexes, 47–48
Regional cerebral blood flow, 50–51

Reitan-Klove Sensory Perceptual Examination, 120–121
Reliable Digit Span, 190
Renal failure, 12
Repeated concussions, 23
Residual schizophrenia, 33
Reversible causes, 14
Rey Auditory-Verbal Learning Test, 142–143, 189–190
Rey Memory for 15 Items Test, 187–188
Rey-Osterrieth Complex Figure Test, 111–112, 147
Risk factors for stroke, 6
Rivermead Behavioral Memory Test, 150
Rooting reflex, 15
RPM. *See* Raven's Progressive Matrices

S
Schizophrenia, 31–35
  episodes, 34
  subtypes, 33
Seizures, 25–29
  drugs, 26
  emotional stress, 26
  environmental stimuli, 26
  fever, 26
  generalized seizures, 28–29
  generalized tonic-clonic seizures, 29
  hallucinations, 28
  hormonal changes, 26
  hyperventilation, 26
  International Classification of Epileptic Seizures, 26–27
  partial seizures, 26–27
  sensory stimuli, 26
  sleep deprivation, 26
  temporal lobe personality, 28
  trauma, 26
Selective Reminding Test, 144–145
Semicoma, 79
Sensation, tests of, 46
Sensory loss, 10
Sensory stimuli, 26
Sexual history, 68–69
Short-term memory, 92
Simple recognition, 107–108
Single-photon emission computerized tomography, 41, 51

Sixteen-Items Test, 188
Skull radiographs, 50
Sleep deprivation, 26
Slow-growing tumors, 3
Smoking, 8
Snout reflex, 15
Sorting tests, 157–161
   Category Test, 161
   Color Form Sorting Test, 158–159
   Color Sorting Test, 157–158
   Object Sorting Test, 159
   Vygotsky Concept Formation Test, 159–160
   Wisconsin Card Sorting Test, 160
Spatial abilities, complex visual functions-tests, 108–117
   Bender Visual-Motor Gestalt Test, 108–109
   Benton Visual Retention Test, 109–111
   block design test, 112
   clock drawing, 113–114
   construction tests, 112
   Raven's progressive matrices, 112–113
   Rey-Osterrieth Complex Figure Test, 111–112
   Trail Making Test, 115–117
Spatial memory, 91
SPECT. *See* Single-photon emission computerized tomography
SRT. *See* Selective Reminding Test
Strength, tests of, 47–48
Strokes, 5–6
   middle cerebral artery, 7
Stroop Test, 134–136
Stupor, 79
Subarachnoid hemorrhage, 12
Subdural hematoma, 9
Suicide attempts, 71
Surgery, 70
Swelling of optic disc. *See* Papilledema
Symptom Validity Testing, 188
Syphilis, 13
Systemic lupus erythematosus, 35

T
Tactile functions, 118–121
   discrimination test, 118–120
   Reitan-Klove Sensory Perceptual Examination, 120–121
   tactile recognition, 118–120
Tactile memory-tactual performance test, 147–148
Tactile recognition, 118–120
Temporal lobe personality, 28
Test of Memory Malingering, 190
Thallium, 13
Thyroid disease, 35
Token Test, 129–132
TOMM. *See* Test of Memory Malingering
Tone, tests of, 47–48
Toxins, 13
Trail Making Test, 115–117
Transient ischemic attack, 8, 10
Trauma, 26
Twenty-one-Item Wordlist, 187

U
Ulcerative colitis, 35
Undifferentiated schizophrenia, 33

V
Vascular anatomy, 6
Vascular disorder, 5–12
   aging, risk factor for stroke, 6
   agraphia, 10
   anterior cerebral artery infarcts, 7
   ataxia, 10
   atherosclerosis, 6
   cerebrospinal fluid, 9
   cerebrovascular accidents, 5–6
   Circle of Willis, 6
   contralateral sensory loss, 7
   dementia, 7
   diabetes, 8
   dysarthria, 10
   embolus, 8
   endogenous depression, 10
   expressive aphasia, 7
   Halstead-Reitan Battery, 9
   homonymous hemianopsia, 7
   hypertension, 6, 8
   Impairment Index, 9
   infarcts, 7–8
   ischemia, 8
   posterior cerebral artery infarcts, 7

risk factors for stroke, 6
schizophrenia-like episodes, 34
sensory loss, 10
smoking, 8
strokes, middle cerebral artery, 7
subdural hematoma, 9
transient ischemic attacks, 8, 10
vascular anatomy, 6
vertigo, 10
visual disturbances, 10
vomiting, 10
Verbal fluency, 133–134
  categorical fluency, 133–134
  Controlled Word Association Test, 133
Verbal functions screening, 125–137
  aphasia, 125–132
  Aphasia Screening Test, 126
  naming, 132
  reading fluency, 134–137
  verbal fluency, 133–134
  Wide Range Achievement Test–IV, 136–137
  writing fluency, 134
Verbal memory, 91
  learning problems, 140–145
Vertigo, 10
Vigilance, 85
Visual disturbances, 10
Visual functions, 104–106
  color perception, 105–106
Visual memory, 91, 93, 145–148
  brief visuospatial memory test-revised, 147
  Rey-Osterrieth Complex Figure Test, 147
  tactile memory-tactual performance test, 147–148

Visual recognition, 106–108
  design recognition, 107–108
  face recognition, 107
  figure recognition, 107–108
  Peabody Picture Vocabulary Test–IV, 106
  simple recognition, 107–108
Visual-spatial memory, 93
Vitamin deficiency, 12
Vomiting, 10
Vygotsky Concept Formation Test, 159–160

W
WAIS-R. *See* Wechsler Adult Intelligence Scale–Revised
WCST. *See* Wisconsin Card Sorting Test
Wechsler Adult Intelligence Scale, 193
Wechsler Adult Intelligence Scale–Fourth Edition, 55, 139
Wechsler Adult Intelligence Scale–Revised, 15, 85
Wechsler Adult Intelligence Scale–Third Edition, 190
Wechsler Memory Scale, 91
Wechsler Memory Scale–IV, 148–149
Wechsler Memory Scale–Revised, 16
Wernicke-Korsakoff syndrome, 12
Wide Range Achievement Test–IV, 136–137
Wide Range Assessment of Memory and Learning–Second Edition, 149–150
Wilson's disease, 12, 19–20
  suicide rate, 20
Wisconsin Card Sorting Test, 153, 160, 195
WMS. *See* Wechsler Memory Scale
WRAT-4. *See* Wide Range Achievement Test–IV
Writing fluency, 134